WHY

HEALING

HAPPENS

O.T. Bonnett, M.D.

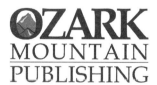
OZARK
MOUNTAIN
PUBLISHING

PO Box 754
Huntsville, AR 72740

www.ozarkmt.com

Library of Congress Cataloging-in-Publication Data
Bonnett, O.T. - 1925 -
"Why Healing Happens" by O.T. Bonnett
A medical doctor of 44 years provides a combative and provocative guide for those who would take charge of their own good health.
   1. Healing   2. Diseases - causes and theories of causation
   3. Alternative Medicine
   I. Bonnett, O.T., 1925 - II. Title

Library of Congress Catalog Number: 2006926106
ISBN: 1-886940-93-2

Cover Art and Layout by www.enki3d.com
Book Design: Julia Degan
Book Set in: Times New Roman, Windsor LtCn BT

Published by

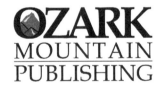

PO Box 754
Huntsville, AR 72740

www.ozarkmt.com
Printed in the United States of America

To my best friend,

RALPH WARNER

SPECIAL THANKS TO MY GUIDE

Anyone interested in having the author conduct seminars
or give lectures on metaphysics or self-healing,
please contact:

O.T. Bonnett, M.D.
P.O. Box 1272
Raton, NM 87740

Telephone: (505) 445-2847
e-mail: BONNETT12345@MSN.COM

Other books by O.T. Bonnett:

Reincarnation: The View from Eternity
What I Learned After Medical School

Publisher's Disclaimer

The cases described in this book are individual and medically specific. Both the publisher and the author assert here that no one under any form of medical care or maintenance should alter his or her regimen without thoroughly discussing any change in diet or medication with a qualified physician.

CONTENTS

PREFACE

TTAINING WISDOM is a gradual process. When students undertake the task of learning medicine or any other subject, their heads do not suddenly open up so that God can pour in wisdom. The acquisition of facts does not imply that one has obtained wisdom. Often, wisdom has little to do with knowledge. So it is with metaphysics. As I acquired metaphysical knowledge, I realized that I needed to integrate it into the basic precepts of medicine. This was an ongoing and endless process that was always exciting and rewarding. Through it, I found myself developing a far broader understanding of humankind, health, and disease. My colleagues' views seemed to me much too constrained, static, and shallow. Medical problems that seemed to confound them often appeared relatively simple and obvious to me when I applied a metaphysical approach.

I constantly hear it stated that the United States has the best health care system in the world. It is so wonderful, some even argue, that there is no need to change it. Although it may be true that the U.S. system of medical care is technically superior to anything else available in the world, it continues to exhibit many serious flaws. For one, there is no incentive in the current system to help people stay healthy. Worse yet, most of today's medical doctors have little training and even less interest in maintaining *health*. On the contrary, doctors wait until illness occurs and then attempt to eliminate it. This is crisis care, not health care, and it is far too costly and ineffective to be supported by tax dollars on a universal national level. The fact that 90 percent of all health care money is spent in the individual's last year of life should give pause in itself. With the present system, patients often receive an inappropriate number of tests, X rays, and other diagnostic procedures when their problems are rather straightforward and simple. Frequently, therapeutic measures are too costly for anyone other than the very wealthy and those on welfare.

As I listen to those who are now proposing new health care plans for the United States, I don't hear them discussing how patients who desire chiropractic, optometric, herbal, or homeopathic care will be included in the proposed "total coverage" packages. Our health care planners have not even mentioned acupuncture, hypnotherapy, or treatment by medicine men. Yet these, too, are proven, valid forms of healing, and those who seek them rather than going to traditional doctors should not be excluded from the package of benefits or forced to payout of their own pockets when others receive subsidized allopathic care. Allopathy is the school of medicine that treats illnesses and injuries by the use of various drugs and surgery. If we are truly a nation that prides itself on freedom of choice, then we should not establish one brand of care as the official national form of medicine any more than we should have an official religion or a single party political system. And so, just what does the government mean by "total coverage"?

In most national health proposals, allopathic medicine is the only form of health care considered, even though it is far from perfect. Truth be told, at times allopathic strategies are wholly ineffective. If the government is going to continue paying for scandalously expensive medicines (many of which do not work), organ transplants, and cardiopulmonary resuscitation out of tax dollars, it should pay for other, often much more effective treatment modalities as well.

This book is written for the lay reader, not the doctor, although I genuinely hope that physicians, too, may find it valuable. To those who object to the concepts and treatment methods I will introduce on the basis that my "proof" is anecdotal, I can only say that the anecdotes are used here to explain principles and not as proof in the scientific sense of the word. Neither will this be a "how-to" book full of exercises or instructions in the ordinary sense of the word. *"Why Healing Happens* is a book of different *concepts. **Exercises and practices do not heal. Concepts heal.*** Nor am I offering a belief system. Enlightened concepts pertaining to the nature of humankind and our role in the universe are what allow us to take conscious, effective control of the healing process.

We are responsible for our own well-being; our health, illnesses, and recoveries. But no individual will understand his or her relationship with health and illness without getting past the thought that guilt or blame plays a role in the process.

In the final analysis, I believe that you will have to lead and entice your doctors into abandoning old, inaccurate formats and beliefs concerning illness and what constitutes proper treatment. But even without their help, applying the concepts and beliefs outlined in this book to yourself and your physical problems will enable you to make great progress in conscious healing. You do not need permission from your physician to adopt the concepts I will outline here. You can do and think these things surrounded by doctors who think otherwise and still gain the benefits of your new understanding. The public can no longer afford to allow members of the medical-industrial complex – the American Medical Association, lawyers, insurance companies, and government – to insert themselves between us and our common sense or to drive a wedge between us and our physicians. Perhaps with this book we can make a start.

PART ONE

CONCEPTS FOR WELL-BEING

CHAPTER ONE

SOME PROBLEMS WITH ALLOPATHIC MEDICINE

THE TELEPHONE RANG. I turned to look at the clock, trying to avoid disturbing two of my cats that were curled around me as I lay stretched out on the bed reading. It was 10 P.M. I lifted the receiver and spoke a husky hello.

"O.T., did I wake you up?" asked the voice on the other end.

"No," I assured him. "I was just lying here reading a bit." I recognized the voice – it was Bill, a friend I had not seen for a couple of years.

"Look," he went on, "I've got this problem, and I want to talk with you about it."

Two years before, I had assisted Bill with a psychological problem through the use of hypnosis. Subconsciously, as is so often the case, he had been dragging old memories and associations into the present – in this case, memories from an earlier life.

He went on without pausing, telling me he had a painful left heel and that the trouble had been diagnosed as a spur. It had been bothering him for the better part of two years and was getting worse. Numerous visits to the doctor had resulted in prescriptions for various anti-inflammatory drugs, heel cups and pads, and two injections of cortisone into the heel. Finally, he had been referred to an orthopedic surgeon who had advised surgery to scrape the calcium from the tendon and remove the spur. Bill's problem was that he didn't have any health insurance, and the surgery and the hospital bill would be about three thousand dollars. He had two thousand dollars, his life savings, in the bank and was trying to accumulate the final thousand. What he wanted from me was advice on anything he might do to relieve the pain until he could have the surgery performed.

"Why do you want to have surgery on your heel? Has anyone explained to you what a heel spur is?"

"I don't *want* surgery, but the surgeon and my doctor both say an operation is the only thing that will help. They say the spur and calcium deposit are causing the pain and until they're removed I'll never be any better. In the mornings, O.T., it's so painful I can hardly walk. It gets a little better as the day goes on, but after I've been on my feet all day, it aches so bad at night I can hardly get to sleep."

"Look, Bill, neither the calcium deposit nor the spur is causing your pain. You have chronically injured tendons where your foot muscles attach to your heel bone. They hurt because they are inflamed, not because of the calcium deposit. Mother Nature has a tendency to deposit calcium in chronically irritated tendons and ligaments. Scraping it out or cutting the spur off will not stop the pain."

"What do you mean? I have an uncle who had his heel operated on by this same surgeon and he's fine." There was a note of irritation in Bill's voice.

4

"Good, I'm glad he got better, but the surgery didn't have anything to do with his recovery – not directly, anyway. If he got well, it was because he believed he would."

"Yeah, yeah, I know you're into that holistic stuff, but not me. I just want to know what I can do right now. I hurt the darn thing a couple of years ago standing on a ladder painting my living room. At first it hardly bothered me, but it's getting worse by the day. Now I'm using a cane and hobbling around like a crippled old man. I can't sleep at night. I'm exhausted. I need help!"

"Come see me," I urged. "Maybe we can work something out. In the meantime, don't have any more cortisone injections. If two didn't make it better, more won't do any good, and if you have more, they may actually cause some damage. And Bill, don't let that guy cut on your foot."

Two weeks later Bill hobbled through my back door, leaning heavily on a cane. As we sat and visited over a few cups of coffee, I noticed he had a bruise on his arm. Finally, I took a look at his heel. It was visibly swollen and exquisitely tender where the long muscles of his arch attached to the heel bone. He had a couple of bruises on his leg as well.

"How much do your gums bleed when you brush your teeth?" I asked.

"What does that have to do with my foot?"

"With all those bruises, I want to be sure you don't have borderline scurvy," I answered. "When you're lacking in vitamin C your body can't heal wounds properly. Do you take any vitamins?"

"Well, my gums do bleed quite a bit, and no, I don't take vitamins. I used to, but my doctor told me it was a waste of money for anyone who ate well to take vitamins, so I quit them about a year ago."

"Your body can't heal itself if it doesn't have the proper materials. And you can't depend on food having all the nutrients you need. Get back on a good multivitamin-mineral tablet, and

5

take at least five thousand milligrams of vitamin C in addition to what's in the multivitamin. Now, let's see what else may be preventing you from getting well."

We went into the living room and I hypnotized him. I knew Bill was a good hypnotic subject from our work the last time. It took only about five minutes to lead him into a deep trance. Then I asked if he had ever injured his left foot before. I told him that he did not have to recall the pain of the injury if one had occurred, only the fact itself. He was silent for a couple of minutes, thinking. Then he replied, "Oh, yeah, I sure did. Three, maybe four lives ago I had my left foot nearly torn off. I was working as a stonecutter in a quarry. A huge slab of stone fell over and crushed my foot against another huge stone. It took them several hours to pry the rocks apart and free my leg. My heel was crushed and nearly torn off. I was a cripple after that, hobbling around with a cane. . . just like now." He smiled.

"Did you ever injure that foot in any other lives?"

He was again silent for a minute or so in deep thought. "Not that I'm aware of," he replied.

While he was still under hypnosis, I informed Bill that his foot was a new one in this life and that it did not have to hurt. Later, we talked about the old injury, and I explained that he might have to continue talking to his heel for some time in order to get its attention. All that inflammation was not likely to disappear overnight. I explained that he should say, "Now we do not need this pain. We have a new foot that has not been injured, so we can forget about that other injury to that other foot. We are fine, and we do not need to be tender, swollen, or painful."

About ten days later I called him to ask whether he had been talking to his foot as I had told him to do. He evaded my question by saying that he had been taking the vitamins as I suggested and that his gums had almost stopped bleeding. Finally, he admitted that his heel was not any better. Again, I told him that it sometimes takes a while to get the cells' attention. I advised him to talk to his heel at least once a day and urged him to use the

6

pronouns "we" and "us" when addressing his foot.

A month later, Bill called me about ten in the evening. I asked about his heel and he began laughing.

"You know, O.T., I have to tell you something funny. When you told me all that stuff about talking to my foot and saying 'we,' I thought I'd never heard such a line of bull in my life. So I didn't talk to it – let alone like you told me to. But after you called me the last time, I got to thinking and said to myself that, in all the years I've known you, you've never said anything that wasn't true. So, after thinking about it for a while, I decided to give it a try. My foot was aching like a son of a gun, so I meditated before going to sleep. I said that *we* did not need the pain, that *we* had a new foot. I said all the things you told me to say. The next morning I woke up, went to the bathroom, and was back in bed before realizing that my foot didn't hurt! There hasn't been a lick of pain in it since. The swelling is gone, and I can push on the spot that used to be sore and there's no tenderness at all. You have to forgive me for doubting you in the first place."

I assured him that he owed me no apology, for he was the guy having all the pain.

What I had told Bill to do flew in the face of what his own doctor and the orthopedic surgeon had told him. In addition, he had been conditioned from childhood to believe that things *happen* to people. That they are *victims* of illnesses and injuries, and that only doctors can make things well with pills and surgery.

This one case is representative of the problems of modern medicine and the need for a change to a more eclectic approach. Most doctors of today take a very mechanistic view of medical problems, and do the best they can within the constraints of their belief system. Bill's doctor had made the correct diagnosis: that the tendon was inflamed from the injury caused by standing on the ladder. And he did all the proper things, according to the accepted practices of his profession. He prescribed anti-inflammatory drugs in the proper dosage and then, upon their failure, injected corticosteroids, which have a more powerful anti-inflammatory effect. When this method proved ineffective, as had the heel cups and all the rest, he referred his patient to a surgeon as he had been trained to do – all very proper, accepted stuff.

Surgeons are trained to operate on people. If you see one with a complaint and keep going back often enough, you are almost certain to end up having an operation of some sort. All people perceive things according to their training and experience, and doctors are no different. Internists see medical problems as infections or as the result of some physiologic or metabolic defect, and so they try to think of what medicine will alter the process. Surgeons see diseases, growths, and illnesses as potential reasons to do surgery. As the old adage has it, from the perspective of a hammer, all the world is a nail. Doctors behave in the same fashion. They have been trained to do so. Orthopedic surgeons are a lot like carpenters; in fact, they even joke about it. They are trained to see human bodies as a collection of broken parts in need of repair. They approach broken bones as if they were structures to be rebuilt. The good ones know that if it is possible to set a fracture without surgery, the patient is better off. In other situations, they make repairs using pins, screws, and plates. Upon seeing the heel spur and the calcium deposit in the tendon of my friend's foot, the surgeon immediately perceived things that were not supposed to be there. He felt obligated to remove them. *But sometimes patients get better after surgery, and sometimes they do not.*

If Bill had undergone the surgery, there was a good chance that he would not have gotten much better, because his original problem would not have been addressed. As you will see through the concepts presented in the following pages, if surgery had been successful in relieving Bill's pain, it would have been due to his believing. And, therefore, the cellular consciousness of his heel tendons believing that a cure had been effected due to their cooperation with the treatment. It would not have been because of what the surgeon actually did. Certainly, the original strain that had resulted from standing on the ladder rung had long since had time to recover. In fact, Bill had said that it wasn't very sore at the time of the original injury. Once it started, however, it got progressively worse. From my perspective, "being involved with that holistic stuff", as Bill described it, the fact that his heel continued to worsen over time indicated that something was going on within his psyche.

Over forty years ago I learned that injuries and diseases associated with other life experiences often result in illness or symptoms in this life. The mechanism resembles a conditioned reflex in many ways. Had I not known this, or had I not had the skill to use hypnosis to ferret out the deeper problem, Bill certainly would have been in for an expensive surgical procedure, the risk of an anesthetic reaction, infection, and all the things that sometimes attend having an operation – perhaps even death. It is possible that he would have limped about for years, perhaps all his life.

Bill was also suffering from malnutrition, which was totally overlooked by his physician. The doctor was obviously unaware of the importance of good nutrition and, what is more, did not recognize the symptoms of scurvy that were staring him in the face. In my opinion, telling Bill to stop taking vitamins was malpractice. It was possible that Bill's foot might have gotten better just from restarting his nutritional supplements – in particular, the higher dose of vitamin C. On occasion I have seen this sort of thing happen. However, Bill needed other intervention.

Bill's painful heel was not caused by the calcium deposit or the spur. It was the result of a psychophysical interaction that perpetuated the inflammation from the original injury of standing on a ladder. For the medical profession to continue ignoring the psychological and perceptual aspects of disease and address every illness and symptom it confronts as a physical event, as something that *happens* to patients, is wrong, shortsighted, and expensive. It may be very profitable for the doctors, but it is ruining the economy of the nation and is responsible for bankrupting many families. Worse, many patients are going about ill or hurting when it is unnecessary to do so. In short, we need to accept some broader, more eclectic approach to illness.

Recently, there has been increasing evidence that the public is ready for a change. Bill Moyers's television program, "Healing and the Mind," and more recently a miniseries, "Healing and the Heart," have addressed the subject, but they have only scratched the surface. What needs to be shown is that allopathic medicine, metaphysics, and alternative methods can be melded into a single, highly effective approach to health and treatment. These approaches to health are not contradictory, nor are they equivalent or parallel. Rather, they tend to be totally complementary. Today, a great many books and television programs purport to deal with alternate approaches to medicine, but the vast majority of them fail to deal in depth with the relationship between health and the intent to be healthy. On the contrary, they titillate the imagination, leaving much unsaid, and many times indicate that in some fashion alternative treatments are mysterious. All this in a world where traditional medicine proclaims many alternate approaches dangerous – as though allopathic medical doctors rarely lose a patient.

Time is running out. The United States is on the brink of passing some form of universal health care into law, and if it is patterned after our present form of health care delivery, it will likely bankrupt the country. Allopathic medicine, as it is practiced today, is too expensive to be paid for by a universal government program of any kind. Worse yet, it will not deliver what we hope to receive. In truth, it never has. We have allowed ourselves to be deluded by the glamour of technological tricks such as organ transplants, fancy "Star Trek" gadgets, and the like. As with so many other facets of our lives, we equate toys and fancy rhetoric with creativity and wisdom.

My purpose in this book is to present a new paradigm of disease. Once the new model is explained, I will show how it can augment and enhance what medicine has to offer today. I know already that traditional physicians will not give much consideration to these new concepts. But I'm convinced that the new paradigm could revitalize the average medical practice if doctors would only integrate its concepts into the traditional systems.

To begin, let us take a brief overview of where we are today. Americans are living under the delusion that they have the best health care in the world. Although this assessment may be valid from certain points of view, it is totally inaccurate from many others. If you insist on having an organ transplant, coronary artery surgery, or some other equally exotic mechanical procedure, there is nowhere better to be than here. But for treating simple, everyday illnesses, we have one of the worst health care systems imaginable. Doctors run many tests, do many procedures, and prescribe many medicines that are both unnecessary and expensive. Frequently, today's medical care does not deal with minor problems appropriately, and it is not available to many among the middle class and the poor.

The medical profession has a tendency to treat every problem as though it were life threatening. It does not properly distinguish between minor health problems and medical catastrophes. Physicians continue to consider patients as victims of disease, and patients subscribe to the same concept. As a result, nearly all medical efforts are aimed at "fighting" illness after it has occurred. Rich and powerful institutions have arisen on the basis of this false principle: humankind pitted against cancer, against muscular dystrophy, against heart attacks, against arthritis, against AIDS, against mental illness, against this, against that. As a nation, we spend our resources and energies *against* everything.

Doctors perceive illness in a totally different way than do non-physicians. In our training, we doctors are taught to see illness as a set of general processes. We are not expected to view a case as a singular process within an individual human being. Except in situations in which the behavior of the patient was directly responsible for the development of the disease, such as emphysema or lung cancer caused by smoking tobacco, doctors do not think of the patient as having any real connection with the illness other than as its hapless victim. Oddly, even in those situations, we turn right around and talk about "victims" of lung cancer and of the tobacco industry rather than the cancer being the result of the individual's *conscious* choice to use tobacco.

Of course, not all patients view illness in the same way. In her essays *Illness as MetaPhor* and *AIDS and Its MetaPhor,* Susan Sontag does a masterful job of describing the way society and individuals look at disease. She points out that, in the last century and the first part of this one, tuberculosis was the disease to be feared, much as cancer and AIDS are now. Society, however, did not shun the bearers of TB; rather, it glorified them. The wan, pale look of the tubercular individual was thought of as romantic, even attractive. TB was the disease of poets and philosophers. Healthy people tried to mimic the sallow, hollow-chested look of one dying of the disease. Having tuberculosis was not considered shameful. It was to be admired – even envied.

Sontag goes on to say that today, in contrast, the person with cancer is thought of as somehow unclean. Too often the disease goes unmentioned. Frequently, the doctor even conspires with the relatives to keep the diagnosis from the patient. In recent generations, cancer has been synonymous with death. AIDS has the same connotation, with the added onus of contamination and sin. Cancer and AIDS have no such romantic metaphors as TB enjoyed. On the contrary, cancer is viewed as the invasion of the body by cells that have run amok; AIDS, as an affliction that comes from some unholy contact.

Let me address the first criticism that will be leveled at this book. Accepting a new model for illness may seem to imply accepting blame for being ill. Sick people reading this book may worry that the cause of their illness lies in some guilty or harmful wish they've internalized. "Isn't it bad enough that I am a victim of this illness," they may think, "without being told that I am to blame for getting sick in the first place?" It is not the intent of this book to place blame on anyone. On the contrary, ***through the process of accepting that you have had an active role – however unconscious – in the development and creation of a disease or injury, you empower yourself to heal yourself.*** The model I will present here is not my own invention. I did not make it up. It is the way things actually are. Anyone who is willing to spend some time thinking about the dynamics of this model for disease will recognize its validity. Truth should not hurt anyone. If we are hurt by hearing the truth, then we must reevaluate our position as human entities. In this case, the old adage "the truth will set you free" could not be more accurate.

Traditional medicine's attitude toward alternative methods is suggested by the following metaphor. Assume it is the practice for everyone to drive along the shoulders of the road and in the ditches, where there are all sorts of broken bottles, trash, and nails. Suppose that drivers do so because everyone has always been *instructed* to drive in the ditches and stay off the pavement. Eventually, every car develops flat tires or front end damage, and has to be hauled in for repair. Everyone accepts driving in the ditches and having flat tires, wheels out of alignment, and occasional broken axles as normal. And so it goes, for generations.

Over time, "professional proper mechanics" arise for the purpose of telling you how to avoid trouble while driving in the ditches, and the importance of calling them when your car is damaged. To become one of these experts, these PPMs, an individual has to attend a special school to learn how to categorize the damage based upon whether it was caused by a nail, a broken bottle, or a rock. PPMs also learn to repair the damage. But any mechanic who suggests driving on the pavement is branded a quack or a cultist. The PPMs continually try to run the others out of business – for the public's own good, of course – and threaten that they will not be responsible for the consequences if people start driving on the pavement.

No driver is to *blame* for driving in the ditch, for to take any other course would have made him or her appear. . . different. People drive in the ditches because they've never been taught how to reach the pavement, and because those who do break away and drive on the pavement are discredited when they report fewer flat tires.

To begin our travels, we must first have the desire to leave where we are, have a destination for which to aim, and enough confidence in ourselves that we are equal to the trip and the challenge. If we are brave enough, we just might find that driving on the pavement really does lead to fewer flat tires. As I look about me at the various people who inhabit my world, I find that, in some way and to some degree, nearly all of them are worried about their health. Perhaps this is to be expected. The newspapers, magazines, and television are full of horror stories about this or that illness. If the articles are to be believed, everything we do or eat, or do not do or eat, places us at some risk. On further analysis, it appears that the vast majority of these frightened people have no sense of a psychological center. They lack an understanding of their purpose as human beings. As children, few received instruction concerning life goals, the importance of living with honor, or how to take command of their lives. Many were given lots of rules, but laying down rules is not instruction. This observation caused me to sit back and think about the people I have known who have led well-centered lives and are healthy, vigorous individuals. From my forty-four years of medical practice, I know that the one leads directly to the other. Nearly all of the most vigorous people I can bring to mind have had a clear grasp of the meaning of life and of their relationship to the Universe. Few have been deeply into metaphysics, but all have possessed an innate understanding of what living is about. In short, I believe it is critical that every human being have some grasp of the infinite if he or she is to live as a whole and healthy person.

If we are going to shift toward a different paradigm of

disease and illness in order to improve health, we must adopt new concepts of the nature of humankind and the Universe. Without some comprehension of metaphysical truths and nonphysical explanations for illness, the different model will not make any sense to anyone. So, with the new model for disease that I offer here, I will need to introduce you to some new models for living as well.

The new model is simply a different way of looking at disease and trying an alternate approach to healing. It is not untested or untried. It is just not tried often enough, and it certainly cannot be thought of as a standard, conventional approach to therapy. However, if we do not intend to drive in the ditches of life forever, I suggest that there is no better time to reinstruct the reflex systems by which we relate to the environment and to ourselves.

CHAPTER TWO

A PREMATURE COMMITMENT TO REALITY

WHEN SOMEONE OFFERS a new idea as a cure-all for the troubles of society, I, for one, am a bit skeptical. Far too often such a person is selling something or has an ax to grind. So let me say up front that the concepts in this book concerning a different model for disease are not new; neither are they a panacea. However, when combined with all the tools medicine has at hand today, these concepts are far more effective than modern medicine alone. Many of the ideas and beliefs of holistic medicine have been around since humans first entered the scene and have been quite consistently effective over the ages. The "in" thing today is to speak of eclectic medicine as being New Age. The difficulty is that for too many people the term "New Age medicine" brings up visions of black boxes with flashing lights, sitting cross-legged intoning unusual sounds, olive oil massages, exotic incense burning on little stands, candlelight, crystals, and coffee enemas.

What I will introduce here has nothing to do with such magic; these are not the sort of healing techniques that the average person of this culture can accept. When they are effective – and sometimes they are – it is because they have focused the intent of the individual on health and healing. The proponents of these creative techniques are no doubt sincere, but none of their practices fits into any new model for healing that the whole of the population can embrace, at least not at this time or in this country.

These statements are not to be construed as a denial of the value of acupuncture, chiropractic, homeopathy, herbal medicine, and other approaches to healing, for there are many skilled and successful practitioners of those treatment modalities. All one has to do to become convinced of this is to read Dr. Andrew Weil's latest book. The problem is that over the years the medical profession – the allopaths – have created a void by their closed-minded attitudes. When allopathic methods fail, most doctors refuse to entertain other approaches to healing or to suggest to their patients that they seek someone skilled in other systems. To make matters worse, a number of poorly trained charlatans have attempted to fill the void and have given alternative medical approaches a bad name. Remember, the term "alternative medicine" implies that allopathy is the correct, accepted approach and that other methods are in some way inferior or untrustworthy by virtue of their being different. Before China opened its doors to the West, the Chinese considered allopathy to be alternative medicine, and herbal cures and acupuncture were the standard practices. So, while ignoring the antics and bogus claims of the charlatans, let us make certain that we honor the legitimate practitioners of "alternative medicine," regardless of the field in which they work.

From its inception in 1847 to the present, the American Medical Association (AMA) has been dedicated to the conviction that allopathic medicine is the only valid scientific approach to healing. To stray from the allopathic ranks, therefore, has been tantamount to professional suicide. For years, the AMA kept a stranglehold on every medical doctor. To criticize another doctor, even one who had contributed to a patient's death by sheer stupidity, was judged unethical and reason enough to be drummed out of the organization. For generations, few doctors questioned this position. Fortunately, that is no longer the case.

In the early 1970s, the AMA assessed every member one hundred dollars to help lobby Congress to prevent the development of prepaid clinics and peer review organizations. At that time, I was practicing in a prepaid clinic and served on the peer review committee of both the clinic and the hospital we used. So I thought about their request for a while and, when I had finished thinking, I resigned from the AMA. I wish I had done it years before.

Certainly, other professions have their problems with credibility and exclusion. The other day I saw a cartoon in the paper. Four women were sitting on a park bench. The first said proudly, "My son is a doctor." The next responded with pride that her son was a lawyer. The third lady boasted that her son was a journalist. The last woman said with conviction, "Thank God, I never had any children! "

Out of the confusion, prejudice, hate, name calling, blame, and retribution, something else is emerging in American health care. Gradually, a few more doctors are becoming brave enough to consider less traditional forms of treatment. They are beginning to talk about meditation, vitamins, herbs, and acupuncture. Unfortunately, the public has a tendency to lump everything together under one name and call it New Age. Most people fail to understand that the change consists of little more than learning and rediscovering approaches and therapy that have been around for thousands of years. If we must give this approach a name, let us think of it as it really is – far from being New Age, it is ancient.

Generations ago, doctors began to think that the smidgen of knowledge and skill they had accumulated within their frame of reference was all encompassing. They took the position that everything beyond the boundaries of their belief system was worthless. Physicians peeked through the knothole in the wall of their technology and declared that their limited view was all there was. This was the kind of thinking that inspired the Moslems to burn the library at Alexandria in 641 AD in the belief that no worthwhile knowledge was to be found anywhere except in the Koran. Even now, most practitioners adhere to the conviction that everything worth knowing about medicine and disease is taught in the allopathic medical schools and printed in a few accepted journals. Too many of them reject out of hand all knowledge developed by other schools of healing.

Let's talk for a moment about adopting new ideas and defending old ones. I have yet to meet anyone who does not have ideas that they feel are important to defend. One person may have strong convictions about politics; another may hold religious beliefs for which he or she bears the same level of devotion. Others may be downright militant about which fly is best suited for catching trout, or what time is best for planting cucumbers. Many of these beliefs are held with a tenacity that defies reason. Problems arise in every field and at every level of human interaction when individuals assume *heavily defended, premature commitments to reality.* Both conflicts and cul-de-sacs develop whenever beliefs or ideas become positions from which the believer refuses to budge.

For example, if a man firmly believes that there is no such thing as so-called psychic healing, no amount of evidence is likely to change his mind. Most likely he will refuse to consider the possibility of being healed by psychic means. Once he assumes his defensive position, he is forever frozen in thought. But it is not necessary to accept the reality of either assumption. All that is necessary is to adopt a *neutral* stance and intellectually toy with the possibility that such things could be true. From a neutral stance, we do not have to defend our position or adopt its opposite. We are free to discuss the concepts, looking at each dispassionately, evaluating their pros and cons. Taking a position is not unlike standing on a teeter-totter to get a better view. It matters little which end of the board one chooses to stand upon, for once a position is taken, one's feet are only a couple of inches above the ground. But, taking the neutral position, standing in the middle with both feet resting comfortably at the fulcrum, one can reach a higher plane and a wider view. True, one will be required to maintain equilibrium, balancing equally with both feet. But, with a bit of practice, stability can be maintained. And from this vaster view, a considered opinion can be formed.

So it is with life and with beliefs. We must constantly assess our belief systems, testing our primary assumptions by taking a neutral stance when faced with new ideas. Doing this helps us avoid becoming rigid and offers constant opportunity for intellectual and spiritual growth.

Years ago, I examined an old belief. During my entire life I had held the opinion that unless an artist painted like Rembrandt or sculpted like Michelangelo or Rodin, he or she lacked talent and was perpetrating a fraud on the public by calling the work art. At a church conference titled "The Shape of the Parish," the then-head of the adult Christian education department of the Presbyterian church, Bill Summerscales, gave a lecture on the history of art, complete with slides. For some reason, it occurred to me to assume a neutral stance and start with the premise that the artists were sincerely attempting to communicate in a different form than had the old masters. Within a few minutes, my eyes were opened to the marvels of modern art. Cubism suddenly made sense and came to life. Picasso's sweeping lines and colors touched me so deeply that tears came to my eyes. I was ashamed of the attitude I had maintained for so many years. And all this enlightenment was accomplished by having assumed a neutral stance.

My quarrel with the medical profession is with the rigidity of its thought and lack of vision. After taking an oath to do everything to help the patient, too many allopaths draw a boundary line around their few dinky facts and attempt to pass them off as a great wealth of knowledge. Having pledged to help the patient, those "traditional" doctors do so only as long as it can be accomplished with the bits of information contained within their limited belief system. Rather than learning from other healing disciplines, such physicians take the attitude of a jealous lover who kills his sweetheart if she looks at another, saying that if he cannot have her, no one can. It is not uncommon for medical doctors to threaten their patients, saying things like, "If you go to a chiropractor, don't bother coming back to me."

The circle the medical profession draws about its collection of facts is not a line drawn in the dust of convention. It is a ten-foot thick reinforced concrete wall that extends upward to the clouds. Once in a while, some physicians may dare to climb to the top of the wall and peek over toward the lush fullness of the real world beyond, the world of inquiry, knowledge, and wisdom. But too often, they retreat back down the wall into the shadows of conformity, afraid to explore the realm outside without Permission to do so. Many physicians are reluctant to embark on intellectual adventures because their training has taken place only within a prescribed, standard curriculum. I am hopeful that this book might serve as a catalyst for them to blaze new trails to wisdom.

I began my professional life in a normal fashion. Born in Salina, Kansas, in 1925, I spent my early years in Kansas and Wyoming. When I was still a boy, my family moved to Champaign Urbana, where I attended the University of Illinois and graduated from its College of Medicine in 1948. After serving a year of internship and two years of general surgical residency in Chicago, I was called into active duty during the Korean War.

Upon my discharge, I began practice in Champaign – Urbana. During this time, I engaged in a full range of general practice: obstetrics, general surgery, pediatrics, and adult medicine. While doing surgery, I investigated the idea that patients could hear even under general anesthesia, giving them suggestions during surgery to affect their postoperative recovery. I published a paper on the excellent results of these efforts. Working with a friend who was an optometrist, I developed a visual-motor-perceptual training program for dyslexic and "retarded" children who had visual and perceptual problems. Together, we were successful in getting twenty-some children out of specialized education classes, back into regular classes, where most of them became top students. In the early 1950s, I learned to use hypnosis to help many patients recover from "untreatable" illnesses. During the course of using hypnosis, I learned much about how the mind and body interrelate. All this is recounted in detail in my book *What I Learned After Medical School.*

In 1970, I left solo practice and joined a prepaid group practice in Bellaire, Ohio. There I confined myself to general adult medicine. I was the chief of the department of medicine, which was composed of nine other physicians who were either board-certified internists or family practitioners. I was also active on the quality assessment and peer review committees of both the clinic and the hospital where we practiced. During this time I conducted a study on the treatment of heart attacks using a highly effective but controversial approach developed by Dr. Demetrio Sodi-Pallares. Under this regimen, the mortality rate of my patients with heart attacks was reduced to one-third that of patients who received standard therapy. I published a paper on this subject as well. During those years, I became interested in chiropractic and kinesiology and combined many chiropractic treatments into my practice.

In 1987, I left direct practice to take a position as medical director of the hospital in Raton, New Mexico. I retired in June 1992.

Today, we are fully caught up in the worship of "science." We hear that science did this and science did that. News commentators talk about science solving one problem or another. We look to science to find a cure for cancer, AIDS, birth defects – literally everything. We are so caught up with the idea of scientific method that we have become reluctant, even afraid, to trust our own observations, and too often we feel it necessary to turn to an expert or some scientific study for validation.

The situation reminds me of the old story about the man browsing in an antique shop who became intrigued with an ancient instrument. He asked the antique dealer what it was. "It's an old barometer," the dealer replied.

"What does it do, and how does it work?" the customer asked. The dealer had no idea how the thing worked. But, not wishing to appear ignorant, he replied, "It tells you if it's raining. You hold it out the window and then bring it back inside. If it's wet, then you know it's raining."

"But I don't need a barometer to do that," the customer responded in confusion. "I can hold my hand outside and tell the same thing."

"Oh, yes, I know," the dealer replied, "but that would not be scientific. "

I have seen doctors completely discount their personal experience because it conflicted with some article they read. They are so enamored of the scientific method and double-blind experiments that these are all they trust. Often, patients tell of symptoms and reactions that are not reported in the literature or in textbooks. Their physicians, learned as they are in conventional medical wisdom, often discount these reports. Certainly, anecdotal information is not always reliable, but it should not automatically be ignored. In fact, as you read this book, you may find that such an attitude is unwise, *given the fact that we are, to a great extent, the creators of our illnesses.*

Scientists are not always scientific. Far too numerous are examples of scientific observations that are found to be less impersonal and objective than they are made to appear. Almost every month, some news article surfaces that exposes deception and dishonesty in some drug company, medical research project, or manufacturer of medical materials and equipment. Some years ago, *Science* magazine, one of the most prestigious scientific publications, uncovered a case in which several professors from a celebrated university had accepted federal money to fund a fake research project. They wrote a bogus scientific article complete with tables of data that had never actually been gathered.

"Science" has done nothing and never will. It is only a method of investigation people use to test the accuracy of certain assumptions. It is *people* who do things and learn things, sometimes by the use of scientific methods. On many occasions, scientific methods are no more accurate or valid than personal observation, such as in the story of the man with the barometer. Scientific inquiry is based upon the collection and analysis of data and nothing more. Scientific methods of examining and searching for truth are not appropriate for investigating philosophical or metaphysical subjects – or the personal experiences of men and women. *Science is wrong when it limits the validation of personal experiences only to instances it can already explain.*

Beyond this, we suffer a tendency to confuse the acquisition of data with the possession of wisdom. Wisdom lies beyond the accumulation of data. It is, rather, an awareness of the true meaning of facts and of the truth from which they spring. Scientific inquiry and the collection of valid data often rely upon the concept of cause and effect – which is, strictly speaking, never observable. The diligent investigator will eventually discover that certain "effects" always seem to follow certain causal actions. She administers a chemical and the cell behaves differently. But, however long and closely she looks, she cannot see all the forces that bring on the event she has called "effect." She cannot take into account the unseen or unknown forces that may have a bearing on the outcome. Thus, "cause" in the idea of cause and effect is simply an assumption. There is no absolute way to determine whether a sequence of individual events is truly related or not.

This is a book of philosophy – metaphysics – as it applies to the maintenance of health and the development of healing. Metaphysics is, of course, a philosophy that seeks to explain the nature of being or reality. This book will hinge upon the premise that the Universe is capable of perceptions and feelings and is, in a very real sense, cooperative. My purpose here is to introduce new concepts concerning health and non-health. By understanding that we exist in a living Universe and are part of it, we can come to grasp how we produce our illnesses through our beliefs and, equally, how we can heal ourselves through accepting different beliefs. Thus, we can come to accept illness and injury as opportunities to learn. We can embrace these personal difficulties as stimuli to reevaluate our lives and our core beliefs. Once the new concepts I will describe become part of your core belief system, then vast strides in your healing can be accomplished.

Understanding our nature leads to greater success in achieving and maintaining health. When he was in the Nazi death camps, Viktor Frankl observed that those people who could find some existential reason to live nearly always found a way to survive. In the same manner, if we understand our relationship with the Universe and the nature of our being as human entities, we will find ways to apply those principles to our health, our illnesses, and our injuries. The entire purpose of individuated human consciousness is to attain wisdom and to participate in the overall wisdom and creativity of the Universe. To the degree that we do attain wisdom, we can and do participate. The attainment of wisdom requires the assimilation of a mass of experience. Experience is not the same as knowledge. One can experience an event without having any knowledge of what is going on. For example, one can be burned and experience the pain without any knowledge of thermodynamics, but knowing about thermodynamics is no substitute for the experience of being burned.

At some time, in some way, we will experience illness and learn to overcome it. Wisdom cannot be taught, nor can we learn about health and wellness as we would learn mathematics or geography. Buddha, in the novel Siddhartha was thought to have said that knowledge can be taught, but not wisdom, and that the wisdom a wise man attempts to impart always ends up sounding foolish. In the delightful book *The Tao of Pooh,* by Benjamin Hoff, Pooh remarks that Rabbit has a lot of brain and that Rabbit is smart. To this the narrator agrees. Pooh thinks a bit and then observes that this must be why Rabbit never understands anything.

Members of the medical profession have been caught in the same snare of delusion. One of their greatest problems is that, like Rabbit, many allopaths have become impressed with their technological cleverness and their meager collection of facts. They remain confused, equating knowledge and wit with wisdom. They have become addicted to the abundance of medical technology with which they play daily, fiddling with human lives as if they were only Tinkertoys.

Doctors usually hold themselves apart from, and superior to, the rest of humanity. If this is not a true statement, then the stance and the demeanor of members of the profession belie their real attitudes. Physicians who do not want to be branded in this way had best make some effort to correct their image. Physicians must look at their patients as people. They should read something other than their medical journals, for the answers they need are not to be found there. Doctors should look at their failures as indications of flaws in their basic belief system, not as the result of a particular procedure, an unordered test, an unprescribed drug. In short, physicians – and their patients – need to open their eyes to a different view of health and healing.

CHAPTER THREE

AN OVERVIEW OF MODERN MEDICINE

ILLNESS WILL NEVER BE ELIMINATED, nor should we wish it to be. To do so would be like standing in a spring meadow graced with a profusion of wildflowers hoping that it will never rain again. Illness is one of the paradoxes of life, for the two seem at odds with one another. The truth is that illness serves a great purpose. It's a window of opportunity for the spirit – an opportunity to learn and become wise.

Becoming ill may get your attention if you have been working too hard and not taking care of yourself. In a literal sense, your body may be saying, "Give yourself some time to reflect on life. Take some time to be with your family, for you can't sustain this pace forever." A mild heart attack, or the flu, can actually serve as a wake-up call to alter your life pattern, to reassess your priorities. The person who is unaware of the relationship of illness to spiritual development will see the illness only as something that happened to her. She will view herself as just another victim of heart disease or the flu epidemic.

An accident or illness that is potentially fatal may force a decision at a deep subconscious level: whether to fulfill life's purpose or to release oneself from the effort. At these times, illness may become the event by which we close the door on what may well be a single chapter of life. These are things we all must learn to appreciate, and these lessons are equally true for the members of the healing professions.

As I progressed through school and medical training, I felt very much an outsider. When I finally entered private practice in 1952, I was forever aware that one part of me was questioning the medical profession itself. I wondered why medicine was practiced the way it was. Why did people really become ill? Why did doctors assume the attitudes they did? Why were they so narrow in their thoughts and beliefs? I knew that the medical information we were taught, and upon which every other doctor I knew based his or her practice, was superficial and often inaccurate and meaningless. I had this haunting feeling that, despite what appeared to be marvelous results at times, doctors were not touching the real issues. We were like children enthralled with an ornate, colorful bag who never look inside to find the real treasures it contains. I was impressed with the advances that medical research had made, but I knew that there was more to be found by taking an in-depth, metaphysical view that none of my colleagues seemed much interested in exploring.

So I watched and learned. In addition to reading the usual medical literature, I read journals from other disciplines, such as *Science* and the *Journal of Experimental Biology and Medicine.* I read books on neurophysiology, neurological development, educational psychology, and other subjects. In publications such as these I gathered much information that I was able to carry into my practice. What I learned altered my interaction with and treatment of my patients, and I almost always found the resulting different methodologies to be beautifully effective. When they were not effective, they certainly were never harmful. Often I was able to help patients with these alternate techniques when standard, accepted treatments had proven to be of little or no benefit.

Sometimes I tried to discuss these exciting revelations with some of my colleagues and encouraged them to try the techniques as well, but they were invariably uninterested. I thought perhaps it was because their thinking processes were so rigid and constricted that they were uncertain or uncomfortable embracing or even talking about things that lay outside their accepted belief system. I can remember the blank look on their faces when I spoke of some of the things I had learned. I realize now that they had no apperceiving basis upon which to comprehend a single thing I had told them. In short, they did not have a clue what I was talking about.

In addition to the scientific material, I read philosophy and metaphysics, Emerson's essays, the writings of Plato and of Lao Tzu. I was particularly intrigued with Eastern thought. The more I read and learned, the more estranged I became from the so-called mainstream of medicine. It wasn't so much that I thought traditional medical practices wrong, it was that they were so clearly incomplete and were built upon such a narrow, shallow knowledge base. The different stance I developed over those years made the position from which I approached my patients a better one. And that position is not theoretical, for through my experience with the actual application of these principles, I know them to be practical and effective. It is just a different model of health and disease from the one I learned in medical school, and different from that of any other doctor I ever knew. It encompasses most of the scientific methods subscribed to by the medical profession *plus* the means of approaching the mind and the heart of the patient.

From the scientific view, my years in medicine covered many changes in technology and in many aspects of practice. During my internship and residency, our hospital still made its own intravenous solutions and intravenous tubing. We used glass adapters inserted into rubber hoses. These were rinsed out, sterilized, and reused on the next patient. It was very common for the patient upon receiving intravenous fluids to become feverish and develop hives caused by chemical impurities remaining in the equipment. After it became available, we injected an ampule of Benadryl and let the solutions run while the patients scratched. Needles were sharpened by hand on a whetstone, sterilized, and reused many times. Bedpans and urinals made of stainless steel were sterilized and reused. Some doctors were still employing open-drop ether for anesthesia, and a few surgeons were still sewing up bellies with catgut sutures. The hospital laboratories did their tests by hand and mixed their own reagents. Nothing was automated. Major vascular surgery was just beginning to be done with some frequency, and I was privileged to help in the design of some of the vascular clamps that were just coming into use at the time.

In addition to sulfa drugs, we had three antibiotics in those days: penicillin, streptomycin, and tetracycline. We knew it was time to discontinue the streptomycin when the patient started to become deaf. Penicillin allergies were common, and we didn't know that giving tetracycline to children would cause the enamel of their permanent teeth to be discolored. There were no effective drugs to treat high blood pressure and no diuretics other than injectable mercury products. Digitalis-type drugs were the only heart drugs on the market. Hardly ever did we order blood gases on patients. And steroids had not come into use because Hans Selye had yet to publish his book on stress.

The years have brought about a tremendous technical explosion in medicine. Advances in drugs and instrumentation have allowed great strides in what physicians and surgeons can accomplish today compared with what we could do fifty years ago. It is all very exciting and seductive. Every day we hear of some new advance made by scientists. That we have elevated science to the level of a god is not surprising.

I was in the midst of some of these wonderful developments. In fact, I had been promised a place on the surgical team of one of the leading vascular surgeons in the country as soon as I completed my residency. Had I continued, there is no doubt that today I would be doing organ transplants along with all the other surgical mechanics in the field. But a unique psychic experience led me into general practice instead.

I am convinced that every person should go to a family practitioner. Specialists are much too narrow in their approach to illness to properly assume the care of the whole person. Certainly there are things for which family practitioners are not trained. Everyone must know his or her limitations, and that applies equally to specialists. I trained under some of the best specialists in the country, but there were times when I knew they were flying by the seat of their pants. These were the times when they had no one to whom to refer a patient who knew more than they did. No one is capable of doing everything, but I firmly believe that the average family doctor can treat 90 percent of the illnesses that come down the pike as well as, if not better than, the specialist. Keep in mind that nearly all doctors are capable of practicing better medicine than the majority of their patients will allow. At times, the patient dclays his or her own recovery by not permitting the doctor to perform tests or do whatever else is necessary.

The field of general practice offered me the opportunity to learn things I would not have otherwise discovered. It gave me a broader view of my function as a physician, of the profession in general, and of my patients. The problems with which I daily found myself confronted lured me into wondrous and exhilarating adventures of learning. I soon began to discover what I had suspected all along – that the medical profession deals in superficialities. Even today, few doctors wish to be bothered with thinking about the real cause of illness: the beliefs and intent of the patient.

I listened to a panel discussion years ago made up of three editors of medical journals; Linus Pauling, who was a Nobel laureate in chemistry; and a physician whose name I do not recall. The panel members discussed the content of medical journals and, specifically, how papers were selected for publication. The editors admitted that if something was submitted to them for publication that was not mainstream and or did not follow generally accepted principles, they would not publish it, regardless of who wrote it or how well written the article seemed to be.

They gave a number of reasons for their position. First, they did not want to risk publishing something that might later turn out to be less than accurate. Second, they felt that busy physicians needed to read their journals secure in the belief that what they read was standard and accepted. Finally, the three editors all agreed that they did not think the average doctor had the ability to read an article and determine for himself whether it was valid. Dr. Pauling mentioned that some of his research papers had not been accepted by various medical journals. The editors admitted that none of them would have published the papers either, in spite of the fact that they knew them to be well researched, well written, and factual. Pauling's work was considered too controversial.

It is true that physicians' education leads – in spite of their high degree of training – down one narrow path of conceptual thought. Their knowledge is confined to such a rigidly defended area that most have neither the information nor the wisdom to pass judgment on an article containing really new material.

Physicians, as a group, tend to be very impersonal. Perhaps the majority of them don't know how to consider their patients as persons. These are the doctors who think of their patients only as cases: a gallbladder, an ulcer, and so on. A board-certified surgeon I knew some years ago had a big practice. One of the things his patients remarked about him was how kind and considerate he was to them. As we eventually became better acquainted, we often assisted one another in surgery, and on two occasions I treated him in the hospital as a patient. The closer I got to him, the more I realized that he was little more than a consummate actor. My impression was that he did not perceive his patients as persons. He had learned the right thing to say, the right tone of voice, and how to act as if he were concerned. But inside, he was a cold fish, and his main reason for wishing his patients to get along well was that a bad result would reflect on his reputation. Without his good reputation, his income and his ego would be affected.

In medical school, we were cautioned to keep our distance and not become emotionally involved with our patients. In order to maintain our objectivity, we were told to remain aloof from their feelings and not to become immersed in their personal lives. Inquiry into the family history was limited to little more than listing the diseases considered to be hereditary that the relatives may have had, and the number and age of the children. Nobody ever considered asking the patients if they were happy, or delving into any emotional aspect of their lives. If doctors had allowed themselves to see their patients as fellow human beings, it would have been difficult for them to be the kind of individuals most of them were. Of course, I knew some very dedicated, selfless doctors who truly cared for their patients as friends and did everything humanly possible to treat them with all the skill and knowledge at hand. But, unfortunately, doctors of that type seem to be in the minority.

As years passed, I came to realize that the physician who is not aware of his patients' beliefs, fears, hopes, and desires is not very effective as a healer. Medical training primarily involves memorization of sets of facts, and leads the majority of doctors to practice medicine by rote. They learn a certain block of information in their training and simply apply it to each situation as it presents itself. There are few instances in which the medical student or doctor is actually required to reason. What passes for thought is the accurate recall of appropriate data and information previously committed to memory. In general, what they learn is rigidly compartmentalized in carefully guarded mental cubicles. When I was in practice, a condition, situation, or piece of information that was obviously relevant in the broad context of health was seen by most of my colleagues either to fit into a specific medical complex or to be irrelevant. There was little desire on their part to understand why a treatment actually failed or succeeded. If, for example, a patient failed to recover from an infection, they assumed it was because they had not used the correct antibiotic. It never occurred to them that poor nutrition or the patient's intent or belief might have had an effect on her recovery. Instead, most of my colleagues sought simple answers to superficial questions and utilized standard forms of therapy that were approved and accepted by the profession whether they were effective or not.

One outstanding example of the automatic way medicine is practiced by many doctors is illustrated in this chilling true account of an event that occurred about forty years ago. A middle-aged doctor who had practiced in a small Illinois town for many years suffered a mental breakdown and was hospitalized. There it was found that he had suffered extensive brain damage as the result of years of heavy drinking in combination with the abusive use of sedatives. The frightening thing was that IQ testing revealed that his substance abuse had left him severely mentally deficient. There was no way of determining how long he had been getting by, simply passing out pills for the symptoms presented to him by his patients. During a review of his records, it was found that if the patient failed to become better after a few visits, the doctor simply referred her to a specialist. As a result, the specialists in the area all thought he was a wonderful doctor, for he was such a good source of referrals.

Another example of this tunnel vision on the part of physicians occurred several years ago. A board-certified internist of my acquaintance was treating a woman for itching. She was diabetic, and he concluded that she was allergic to the form of insulin she was taking. She had seen the doctor on a number of occasions while he fiddled around changing insulins. One day, a woman friend went to call upon her. At first glance the friend noticed that she was extremely jaundiced. She asked the patient when she had last seen the doctor and learned that it had been the day before.

"Didn't he look at you?" the friend demanded. She suggested the woman see the doctor again that day and insist that he put the chart aside and look at her instead. The woman did as her friend suggested. Shaken out of his usual mode of behavior by her demand, the internist finally noticed her most obvious symptom. Further tests revealed the woman to have an obstructive jaundice secondary to a cancer in her pancreas.

All physicians want to see their patients recover, but an alarming number, like my surgeon friend, want those good results primarily because a lack of success will affect their reputation and in turn their income. As years passed and malpractice suits became more commonplace, doctors became increasingly motivated by their fear of a lawsuit. Much of what doctors do today is defensive in nature, designed to protect them should they be sued, and has little to do with making an accurate diagnosis or helping the patient recover.

Perhaps even more than a lawsuit, doctors fear being labeled nonconformist by their peers. This factor alone prevents many from trying alternative approaches to medicine when it is obvious that the accepted methods are of limited or no value.

To make matters worse, most medical research is aimed primarily at obtaining just a few more quick answers – various physiologic knobs and switches that can be tinkered with through some drug yet to be developed. Over the past several decades, none of the wonderful discoveries touted in the medical literature and on the evening news has had much to do with *why* people become ill or how one might prevent illness. We know already that if, for instance, a patient develops pneumonia or some other infectious disease, it is not simply because she has been exposed to another person who has the infection. *Pneumococci, along with numerous other disease-causing bacteria, can be cultured from the throats of most perfectly healthy people who never develop the diseases.*

Even during the influenza epidemics, I became ill only twice in all the years I practiced, and each time I was under great emotional stress. I never took flu shots myself, yet I was coughed and sneezed upon by patients with the flu fifteen or twenty times a day. Most doctors would tell similar stories. Shouldn't medical research devote considerable resources – perhaps as much as half the total – to discover why people become ill, rather than only searching for methods to help after illness has occurred?

Doctors have always professed an interest in preventive medicine; however, this is just a platitude, repeated by physicians who still have no real concept of what that means. History is filled with examples of dedicated physicians being persecuted by their colleagues for trying to develop ways to keep people healthy. Ignaz Semmelweis was persecuted for his attempts to prevent women and infants from dying as a result of infections incurred during childbirth. He published a paper stating his beliefs in 1860 but was ridiculed by his colleagues, nonetheless. Louis Pasteur's germ theory of disease was opposed, as was Joseph Lister's antiseptic surgery. Hans Selye's ideas and research in the 1940s concerning stress were not properly accepted. He was not persecuted, but his work was largely ignored by practicing physicians. Demetrio SodiPallares' method for treatment and prevention of heart attack were, and still are, belittled despite the fact that they are superior to anything else available today, including all forms of surgery. Linus Pauling was mocked and verbally assaulted for saying that vitamin C could help prevent colds and suppress the growth of cancers. Any doctor today can tell you that if he or she becomes truly involved in preventive medical procedures, teaching their patients about nutrition, prescribing vitamins, using low-salt diets for high blood pressure and heart disease, and other modalities directed at keeping people healthy, they run the risk of being labeled a bit strange by their colleagues.

Over the years, as I increasingly looked beyond the physical cause-and-effect formula to find answers for existential and medical problems alike, I began to realize that the major thrust of medicine and medical research adopted the wrong priorities from the start. There is nothing wrong with identifying disease germs or finding antibiotics that will kill them. Certainly, that is a good thing. There is nothing wrong with learning what we have about physiology and developing medicines to alter body chemistry toward normal. No one would deny the benefits afforded by the diagnostic testing techniques developed in recent years or the technical wonders of surgery available today. The huge error lies in assuming that this direction of investigation, diagnosis, and treatment is the only correct one, to the exclusion of all others. This fallacy has arisen from our complete ignorance of the nature of the

Universe and of humankind within it. In short, the misunderstanding lies in viewing individuals as separate from the Universe. As though each were a mechanical being, living in the world but not of the world.

From the beginning, medical investigation should have been equally motivated to explore patients' psychic nature and its effect upon their health. Rather than being content with the superficialities of apparent interactions of the body with such things as bacteria and viruses, we should have searched in depth to discover why the body joins forces with so-called pathogens to develop an illness. But to have done this would have required doctors to become thinkers and philosophers – healers, rather than mere prescription writers, test orderers, and scalpel wielders. They would have had to come to grips with their own humanity and that of their patients. Such an approach would have required doctors to be men and women of learning, capable of deductive reasoning, with the ability to integrate their thoughts into a workable and inclusive system.

The present-day attitude of physicians began in the mid-1600s with the philosophy of Rene Descartes, who postulated that matter and mind were unrelated to one another. Before that, scholars had been concerned with *why* the Universe functioned as it did, and with the *meaning* behind various events and conditions. After Descartes, scientists refrained from involving themselves with topics such as purpose or with issues of morality and ethics. From that moment, matter and mind, science and religion were forever separated.

In brief, Descartes argued that nothing could be accepted as valid unless it was proven by mathematics, or scientific method. From this point of view, humankind, plants, and animals became nothing more than pieces of biologic machinery, clockwork with which to tinker, which reduces everything to some mathematical value.

Two hundred years later, Charles Darwin's theory of natural selection made a very neat, seemingly closed, explanation for the biologic variation present on Earth. After some discussion, the theory was, for all practical purposes, universally accepted by the scientific community. A few scientists today do not ascribe to Darwin's theory, but they are generally careful not to let anyone know about it.

In 1860, one year after Darwin published his work, Pasteur published his paper on the germ theory of disease. Five years later, too late to help the wounded of the American Civil War, Lister introduced the principles of antiseptic surgery. All these concepts were focused on, and contributed to, the idea that people were *victims* of diseases *caused* by bacteria and other such contaminants. With this conception, it became "man against the elements," and humankind became obsessed with the fight against the forces of nature. If survival of the fittest was to be the order of the day, then men and women made sure that they would be the victors. With this agenda, few would consider humankind to be part of nature; we are, rather, its potential rulers, granted, as it were, a divine right to exploit and despoil everything and every form of life. Seeing ourselves as separate bits of machinery that arrived on Earth as the result of a genetic accident led us to a decidedly defensive stance. Few ever considered the concept that we are each one with the Universe, much less that we might have sought or produced the illnesses from which we suffered. To think that illness might serve a useful purpose was totally out of the question.

Before the discovery that bacteria could produce disease, epidemics were believed to be due to miasmas – bad air – hanging over a town. Inhaling the vapors of a miasma, it was thought, would induce the illness. Once Pasteur demonstrated that anthrax in sheep was caused by bacteria, the concept of miasmas was generally abandoned, and there was a stampede to identify the germs that were believed to be the cause of almost every illness. As more and more "disease germs" and harmful viruses were discovered, the concept that people "catch" diseases became prevalent. And it persists today. Think of the recent advertisements for antiseptic soap in which the mother is beset by harmful germs lurking everywhere, ready to attack her family. Today, we know that certain people are "carriers" of disease germs, but no one addresses the fact that every healthy person harbors millions of potentially harmful bacteria, viruses, fungi, and yeasts all the time. This fact is generally known, but the medical profession chooses to ignore it in favor of the concept of our becoming "victims" of some organism invading from without.

Sulfa drugs were first discovered in 1908 and came into use in the early 1940s. But the real excitement came in 1932. That was the year Alexander Fleming observed that penicillin mold killed certain bacteria and might be useful as a healing agent. Penicillin came into wide use at the beginning of World War II. After that, the frantic race to discover more antibiotics was on. We finally reached the point where most every common disease bacterium had some antibiotic to kill it. Then, as medical science with its array of antibiotics upset the normal balance of life, other bacteria that had never caused illness changed their behaviors. It was as if the body, upon finding that it could no longer die of common infections, readjusted itself to cooperate with other previously benign organisms.

As I write, there is a scientific symposium of doctors and bacteriologists discussing the very real possibility of future worldwide epidemics caused by antibiotic-resistant organisms. It is now known that resistant bacteria have the ability to share genes with bacteria that have never been exposed to the drugs, thus rendering them resistant as well! This concept is very frightening to a society that has rested comfortably on the false premise that infectious diseases are no longer a threat because of all the antibiotics available.

This invasive concept of illness developed even though, as early as 1796, a German physician by the name of Samuel Hahnemann had formulated a theory of treatment he called homeopathy. According to this theory, if the patient is given minute quantities of some drug or herb that will produce the same symptoms as the illness, the body will respond and counteract the illness. Thus, if a patient had diarrhea, an infinitesimal dose of a laxative was given to stop the attack. As the theory developed further, homeopaths also took into account the lifestyle and personality of each patient when deciding upon treatment.

This explanation of homeopathy is greatly oversimplified but is accurate in broad terms, and it works quite well. The allopaths, the regular M.D.s who were in the majority, had very few drugs with which to treat diseases, so they fought back politically. In 1847, they organized themselves, formed the American Medical Association, and took the position that allopathy represented the only scientifically based school of medical care. Using their influence, they succeeded in getting Congress to support their cause, and with their superior numbers, they gained control of the hospitals and the medical societies. Homeopaths, osteopaths, chiropractors, optometrists, and anyone else who differed with the theories of allopathy were branded quacks or cultists. Associating in any way with one of these "cult" professions was reason to be voted out of the medical society. Furthermore, the AMA required that for a doctor to be granted hospital staff privileges, he or she had to be a member of the AMA. The success of the AMA in defaming the other health care professionals did not improve the effectiveness of the allopaths' methods, but it essentially drove homeopathy underground and made other health professionals appear less than competent in the eyes of the public. Though this began to change in the 1960s, the AMA still maintains a stranglehold on Congress and other government agencies and, therefore, on the health care industry in general.

Under the control of the allopaths, medical treatment has become little more than a counterattack against the ravages of illnesses that remain misunderstood. Research has become a frantic attempt to find "weapons" to fight diseases that strike inexplicably. On the surface, allopathy appears to have been victorious, even though people do not live much longer now than they did hundreds of years ago. In ancient times people lived into their eighties and nineties. Some lived well past one hundred. In eras past, primitive tribes had seers who were the keepers of the wisdom and lived to be ancient. Of course, in those days the chances of an infant's surviving were much less than they are today. There were far more things then that proved fatal to infants, children, and adults alike, thus reducing the probability of living to be ancient. But today, with all the advantages of modern medicine, a person who has reached the age of seventy has a life expectancy only about twenty months longer than a seventy-year-old had in 1850, and this is largely due to better sanitation, housing, and nutrition – not to pills or surgery.

Within the constricted focus of its belief system, the medical profession has made great strides. However, the allopaths' mechanistic approach to the body and its ailments is, I'm certain, doomed to grind to a halt. The reason for this is that the principles behind its narrow focus are basically wrong. Ultimately, to go much beyond where it is today, medicine will have to develop a broader view of humanity. The practice of allopathy is not unlike constructing a building without a proper foundation. It may be possible to erect a building one or two stories high on a foundation of mud and sandstone. It may be a beautiful building with expensive furnishings, thick carpet, and masterful paintings hanging on the walls, but unless the foundation has been correctly laid with reinforced concrete, it will eventually fall, and taller buildings are certain to crumble upon themselves.

Physicians must become involved with life – with the whole living person. One cannot learn much about a live cow by eating a T-bone steak. As a matter of fact, there would be no concept of a cow if all we'd seen was beef displayed in the meat market. To understand cattle it is necessary to study them feeding in the pasture and interacting one with the other. By the same token, if one had never seen or heard of an automobile, seeing one on the display floor would hardly give us a hint of its purpose. There would be no way of determining that it could even run by merely looking at it, taking it apart, and reassembling it. It is only upon getting in one, starting it, and driving it that a full appreciation of that complex machinery called an automobile can be made. To know is to become involved.

In the same manner, it is impossible to learn about the living function of a human being by dissecting a corpse. A dead preserved heart will not beat. A pickled brain does not think. A mouth sealed by death will not tell anything of a person's beliefs, fears, ambitions, hopes, desires, dislikes, loves, or accomplishments, *all of which have an impact upon health.* None of these things can be determined, no matter how completely the brain is dissected, analyzed, or tested.

Further, studying disease tells us little or nothing about health. As a matter of fact, most doctors do not even know what health is, beyond defining it as the absence of disease.

A human being is not an object, a body, or a case. Yet that is how the medical profession – and, sadly, most physicians – has officially viewed the patient. The medical profession remains locked into its mechanistic position of thought even when it has been shown to be wrong and outmoded. Here is a simple illustration. If you are having a problem seeing and go to a medical physician, an ophthalmologist, to have your vision tested, he will approach the problem from a mechanical point of view. This is the same point of view that we all learned in school, that the eye functions like a reflex camera. Doctors are still taught this concept in medical school. You will recall the diagram showing the mechanism of vision in which an image of a candle on a candlestick is reflected into the eye. Light is shown being reflected from the object in space back toward the eye. There it passes through the lens and is shown as a little image imprinted upside down on the retina of the eye. This is exactly what happens in a simple reflex camera. It's a nice, neat idea. But there is a problem: vision does not happen this way.

In 1911, and that is a long time ago, Allvar Gullstrand received the Nobel Prize in medicine for proving that the eye does not work in this fashion. Vision is not a function of the eye. Vision is a function of the brain. The eyes simply act as mechanisms to transmit the light impulses coming from the environment to the brain for interpretation. Every point of light reflected into the eye becomes a diffuse pattern of light on the retina. The person has to learn what that pattern of light represents. Vision is a dynamic process of perception, not a mechanical one.

The ophthalmologist who is testing your vision is troubled by trying to examine this supposed mechanical structure. Being a dynamic organ, the eye is constantly adjusting and reacting to the stimuli it receives. In other words, it won't hold still. To counter this, the medical doctor uses drugs to paralyze the muscles of accommodation and applies some mathematical formula to determine what lens is needed to "correct" the problem. He crosses his fingers and hopes that his result is close to being accurate. Once you receive your glasses, the perceptive functions of the brain are forced to adjust to the new lenses. (Optometrists, by the way, handle visual problems using a completely different approach.) The M.D. is about as successful in giving you the proper prescription as an auto mechanic would be in attempting to adjust the timing of your engine with the motor shut off. The only difference is that your car is a mechanical thing and is incapable of adjusting itself the way your visual cortex can adjust to badly prescribed glasses. This is one of a list of almost endless examples that could be given to illustrate the ineffectiveness of the mechanical approach to medical care.

The presently held concept that humankind is separate from the Universe, and that illness is due to things that *happen* to us, disempowers us and depersonalizes the living processes of our own bodies. A person who is not feeling well goes to the doctor and presents his symptoms. The doctor will listen to his heart and lungs, poke his abdomen, and then start running tests. The history, the examination, and the test results will suggest certain disease processes that will then be sorted out and the most likely one picked as the diagnosis.

Actually, the doctor and the patient often cooperate in the development and organization of an illness. Upon finding themselves unable to cope with life's stresses, or when their lives are constricted and unfulfilling, many individuals experience various physical symptoms. These symptoms are usually taken to the physician as an offering of sorts. Validation of those symptoms by some professional is important to the belief system of most people, since we have been trained for generations that we are incapable of making medical judgments ourselves. If the symptoms offered fit into her concept of a "real" disease, the doctor accepts the symptoms and orders tests and treatment. If the symptoms do not satisfy her, they are rejected, leaving the patient with several alternatives. He can either take his symptoms from doctor to doctor, searching for one who will accept them, or he can go home and produce more symptoms. These in turn will be offered for approval until some doctor is convinced that they "fit" into a recognized disease pattern. The physician will then prescribe drugs to alter body chemistry and make the tests return to normal. After a period of time, the patient usually recovers and the physician is given credit for the cure. What is not recognized by the medical profession is that the symptoms are often a physical representation of a deeper psychological problem that the patient has been unable to resolve. When that is the case, the patient will not fully recover until there is some resolution to his spiritual difficulties, no matter what the doctor does. Occasionally, the original physical problem (the symptoms) may go away as a result of the medicine even when the spiritual problem still exists, but it will usually recur or reappear in some other form.

As it is practiced today, medicine creates almost as many problems as it appears to solve, and the technical advances sometimes lead to further difficulties. Everyone has heard about hospital admissions caused by reactions to medicine. In one very real sense, these are actual diseases orchestrated by doctors. Think about what happens to the individual who goes to the doctor for a checkup when he is healthy. The doctor is trained to look for illness. In my earlier years of practice, I used to pretend that every patient potentially had some obscure, fatal disease it was my duty to diagnose and treat. To this same end, patients across the country are questioned in an attempt to discover symptoms they have not mentioned. Tests are run "on a routine basis," and every slight variation from the norm is investigated. All this is done with a studied desire to find some hidden illness in its early stages. But it is more than a little possible that illnesses may be manufactured in the process of looking for them. Not only do people find themselves being treated for things that did not exist before they went in for their annual physical, but the disease is often created by the body to comply with what it assumes to be a directive from the patient and the doctor.

I know of one family who went to a clinic in Illinois made up entirely of specialists. The father went in for his annual physical and was found to have some pus cells in his urine. He was referred to the urologist, who admitted him to the hospital and "worked him up." He was told that the problem was due to the small size of the opening of the urethra at the tip of his penis. According to the urologist, the small opening was causing an obstruction to the flow of urine, which led to the infection. The patient was subjected to surgery in which the opening was made larger. About three thousand dollars later the doctors were finished with him. Then they counseled the man that a small urethral opening is much more common in women than in men. They convinced his wife to come to the clinic for an examination in spite of the fact that she had no symptoms and had never had a urinary tract infection. Sure enough, she was told that she had a stricture as well. Another three thousand dollars later she was finished with her surgery and was told how lucky she was that the problem had been discovered before she, too, had gotten into trouble. Then the urologist warned the man and his wife that these strictures were often hereditary. Really, to play it safe, he told them, they ought to bring in their twelve-year-old daughter to be checked. Having learned a serious lesson, they changed doctors.

Yet another example: when the first coronary care units were designed and people in the hospital started having constant cardiac monitoring by means of ongoing electrocardiograms, many abnormal heart rhythms were documented. These were treated with injections of various drugs designed to return the rhythm to normal. Many lives were supposedly saved by doing this. Certain abnormal rhythms, such as ventricular tachycardia and fibrillation, were considered to be customarily fatal if they were not treated immediately, and often they were. In fact, treating these rhythm disturbances was the major reason for putting a heart patient in the intensive care unit in the first place.

Then someone designed a portable monitoring system. Patients had their hearts monitored continuously for twenty-four hours while they walked about doing their daily activities. Lo and behold, when the patients returned the tape, it was found that some of them had sustained short bursts of these "fatal" rhythms, which had corrected themselves! Doctors had presumed them to be fatal if they were not treated, yet the patients often failed to report any symptoms, even at the times the abnormalities were occurring. In certain instances these monitorings resulted in the prescription of drugs or the implantation of pacemakers to regulate heart rhythm even when the patient had no symptoms. This practice continues and is always justified on the basis of preventing a catastrophe. Many times I'm certain it is warranted, and many times I'm just as sure it's not.

In the first couple of years following the development of automatic blood chemistry analyzers, more people had their blood chemistries tested than in all the years preceding their invention. What was discovered? More than a few people were found to have abnormal tests without a disease to accompany them. Occasionally, some who were desperately ill had no changes in their blood chemistries at all. For example, on a particular day a person's liver might not be working up to par. If blood happened to be drawn on that day, the tests would be abnormal. The aberrant test results did not necessarily mean that the person was ill, but that was not the way most doctors thought, so the patient was often diagnosed and treated for a disease he or she might not have had. Body chemistry is in a constant state of flux, and the automatic tests revealed this to be the case.

In a sense, drawing and examining a sample of blood is like looking at one frame of a motion picture in which you are seen with your tongue sticking out. The one picture does not mean that you always go around with your tongue hanging out. What you see is accurate, but it may not represent the way you usually look. The automatic analyzers are very helpful, but how badly did doctors do treating patients before the automatic testing came about, when only a few selected tests were ordered? Comparing the mortality rate of specific diseases today with the mortality rate of fifty years ago shows no great difference despite all the tests that are run now.

I conducted a study a few years ago comparing the medical outcomes for patients treated by internists with those for patients of family practitioners. I knew that the internists ran many more tests, resulting in hospital bills almost twice those of the family doctors. I wanted to determine whether running the extra tests made a difference in how the patients fared. The cases were carefully matched as to diagnosis, age, and severity of illness. As it turned out, there was no difference in either mortality rate or the speed at which the patients recovered. The extra tests did nothing to improve the quality of care, but they sure did raise the cost of medical care and hospitalization for the patients of the internists.

Many years ago, when I was doing obstetrics, it was routine to check the fetal heartbeat at regular intervals during labor. Sometimes, the infant was found to be in distress and a Caesarean section was performed. Then the automated fetal heart monitor was developed. Suddenly, there was a rash of C-sections because of fetal distress diagnosed on the basis of the monitoring. Before the inception of the monitor, many of the "problems" would not have been picked up with intermittent listening. But there were essentially no more infant deaths then than now. The new technology has not served to decrease the infant mortality rate to any significant degree, but it *has* been responsible for a tremendous increase in the number of Caesarean sections performed.

Still another example: When I joined the Bellaire Clinic in 1970, we did not have a thoracic surgeon. Occasionally, we would find a spot on a patient's lung or some other pulmonary problem that did not respond to medical management, and we'd refer him or her to a chest surgeon. Some years later, we hired a thoracic surgeon who was exceptionally well trained and an asset to our staff. For the first year, he had hardly any chest cases. Then, gradually, we began seeing more and more chest problems. We found more chest tumors. More patients seemed to require chest tubes. There were more and more legitimate problems requiring chest surgery. In a span of three years, he was busy doing chest surgery all the time. Prior to his coming, the few chest problems we saw resolved themselves without surgery. Our clinic was a prepaid clinic. The surgeon, like the rest of us, was on salary, so performing surgery did not increase his income, it just increased his workload. In fact, the more cases that required surgery, the less we received as year-end bonuses. What was the difference? Did his presence "create" the diseases? I feel that's exactly what happened, and the mechanism will be discussed in later chapters.

Some years ago I read an article in the magazine *Modern Medicine* by a physician questioning the value of some of our therapeutic measures. He cited several pairs of cases. One involved a man who came to his office for a routine annual physical. The chest X ray revealed a small cancer in his lung. He was subjected to surgery followed by radiation therapy. After about one year, thousands of dollars' worth of treatment, and immeasurable worry and stress for him and his family, the man was dead as a result of his cancer. Around the same time, another patient came to him with a cough that he had experienced for close to a year. He had lost a lot of weight but, in general, did not feel too bad. A chest X-ray showed a far advanced cancer of the lung with metastases. Treatment was out of the question. The man died within the month. The doctor calculated that both men had lived roughly the same length of time with their disease. The first one, with all the benefits of modern medicine, had experienced a year of mental anguish and financial loss. The other, not knowing about his cancer until the end, had experienced comparatively little stress and almost no expense.

Another of the doctor's pairs of cases involved men with cancers of the lower colon. In one, the cancer was discovered on a routine examination and resulted in surgery, the loss of his rectum, a colostomy, great expense, worry, and the problems of dealing with his colostomy. He died of his cancer four years later. The other man did not come in until he had a bowel obstruction and metastases to his liver. He refused surgery and died within a week. The doctor estimated from the man's history of bleeding that he probably had had his disease about four years as well. With virtually no medical care, he had avoided much worry, a colostomy, and thousands of dollars in medical bills.

The point is that our system of medical care is geared to do many fancy things, but it does little to prolong life. We are taught that, to ensure recovery from an illness of any magnitude, we must consult a physician. Furthermore, we are told that even minor symptoms may be harbingers of grave illness, making it advisable to run to the doctor for every ache and twinge. In many instances, our attempts to prevent illness simply serve as blueprints for the organization of diseases.

The so-called health care industry is a self-perpetuating, money-gobbling monster. Illness is big business. More people live off each of the specific illnesses than ever die of them. In addition to the doctors, nurses, and hospitals, there are support organizations and businesses that exist solely because of the presence of certain diseases. I am speaking of associations created in response to illnesses such as adult-onset diabetes, multiple sclerosis, ulcerative colitis, endogenous depression, and rheumatoid arthritis. I picked these from a list of many simply because these five diseases are curable this minute at almost no cost with information that is now available. They all are caused by reactions to foods we eat and sometimes to chemicals we ingest in other ways. All that is required to arrest the disease is to identify the offending food or agent and eliminate it. Patients will remain disease free as long as they avoid the food or substance that triggers the disease reaction.

Many doctors have known for at least fifty years that these diseases are curable and preventable by this method, but to date, the so-called mainstream of medicine has not accepted this. Those physicians who are still ignorant of the facts can only blame their not knowing on intellectual bigotry. Most, if not all, of the original investigation of disease development through exposure to foods and elements in the environment was done at Northwestern University in the 1940s by Dr. Theron Randolph. He was ultimately rewarded by being asked to leave the institution on the grounds that his research did not conform to "generally accepted models of disease and treatment."

But times are changing. Increasing numbers of individuals would like to take charge of their lives in ways that have never interested them before. Intuitively, every person knows that health care today is not the panacea it is purported to be. If we truly want to be healthy, we simply have to look somewhere besides the medical profession for *all* the answers. It's not that doctors do not perform a worthy service. The problem is that their approach is so terribly limited and narrow that they miss vast opportunities to be of greater help.

Members of the public desperately want some instruction, some external validation that they are not necessarily victims but, on the contrary, have an active part to play in their health and recovery should they become ill. They wish to understand how illness develops and what they can do about the process.

There may even be physicians like me who are disenchanted with the direction their profession has gone. These patients and doctors are the individuals for whom this book is intended. But we need to look at the problem from more different angles.

CHAPTER FOUR

THE UNIVERSE, HUMANKIND, AND HEALTH

I F WE ARE TO DEVELOP and constantly reevaluate an understanding that embraces a different concept of life, health, and disease, we must have some understanding of the metaphysical aspect of human beings and the Universe and of how they relate one to the other. I am not referring to our belief about medicine, surgery, bacteria, viruses, or organ transplants. What is required is not a new way of viewing these things or deciding when they should be applied or how they fit into a different allopathic approach. I am speaking about a change in the concepts of life and illness, a totally new frame of reference concerning diseases and injuries, how they start and how they heal. If one is to accomplish this, there must be some understanding of the relationship among mind, body, and the Universe. At the deepest level, healing does not depend upon medicine, surgery, herbs, yoga, acupuncture, mantras, or any other "thing" that can be applied, taken, or done. *Treatments do not heal – concepts, beliefs, and understanding heal.*

The acceptance of a new paradigm for healing is likely to demand surrender or, at the very least, modification of some old assumptions. It means rooting out our core beliefs and taking them over to the window where the light is better for a closer look. It may entail rethinking all previously held ideas and cherished concepts of health, regardless of how fond we may be of them. Eventually, to conclude the process, it will be necessary to restructure the old framework to accommodate our new perceptions, fitting them together into a logical, accurate, and practical network of facts and ideas. Occasionally, we may find facets of the previously held framework so faulty that they must be abandoned. But such reassessments should be ongoing in the minds of all who dare to claim intelligence and maturity. This constant reappraisal of doctrines should involve every facet of life, not just beliefs concerning our health. Change has always been an essential function and an ingredient of the living Universe. No individual can call himself wise and think that the ideas and concepts he holds are conclusive and irrefutable.

It is advisable for each of us to bear in mind that our reality is based upon many assumptions that are true *only* from our specific point of reference. One of those assumptions is the concept of a linear time frame. Regardless of how it may appear, this is not the way time actually exists in the vastness of the Universe. There, relative time holds sway in a dimension in which all happens at once – what might be termed an "enduring present" of endless possibilities.

In the course of searching for truths, it is equally essential to understand that windows to understanding often present themselves as paradoxes. Many scientists (physicists, for example) spend a great deal of time and effort attempting to solve paradoxes, to explain them away. But to do so completely negates the beauty of the paradox and its reason for existence. A paradox is a window to enlightenment meant to give us a broader, vaster view of reality. Let me use an example. Rather than endlessly staring at a blank wall in our living room, we can cut an opening in it and install a solid pane of glass. It is a window through which sunlight and heat can pass, and through which one can see, yet the wind cannot blow through it, nor can we walk through the window without breaking the glass. Truly, it does expand our view of reality far more than the limited scene available on a blank wall. The window even adds depth and dimension to the room as we gaze at the garden beyond. But is it an opening, or is it not? The window, like a true paradox, serves its purpose while the questions it raises go unresolved. No one would foolishly spend her life looking at the window frame or the dirt and fly specks on the glass and never look through the window at the garden beyond. But many scientists who spend their lives trying to solve paradoxes using highly creative mathematical equations do just that. Using their approach, we would spend our lives endlessly trying to solve the riddle of how the window can be an opening but not an opening while failing to see the beauty of the flowers in the garden beyond.

A paradox is, of course, a situation in which two seemingly opposing concepts or ideas both hold true. An example of this reality is the yang and yin of Eastern philosophy. The Tai Chi figure is a circle divided by an S-shaped line. One half is black and the other white. In the midst of the black is a spot of white, and in the midst of the white is a spot of black. The overall circular form indicates that the figure is all encompassing. The curved line of division signifies that there is no sharp line of demarcation between two opposite values. The specks of opposite values indicate that each value carries the seed of its opposite.

We humans repeatedly fall into many traps of our own making. One of these is the penchant for taking sides. When faced by seemingly conflicting ideas or beliefs, we feel a compulsion to choose between them, as though truth is an either/or affair. In terms of the earlier metaphor, we feel we must accept the window as an opening or reject it as such because we cannot walk through it. We see the either/or conflict in every stage and facet of our lives. Everything is either good or bad, beautiful or ugly, appropriate or inappropriate, black or white. Rarely do we consider that each side might have something in its favor. Consequently, we fall into the mindless trap that has ensnared the physicists, trying to resolve our paradoxes rather than learning from their contradictions. Individuals who adopt rigid ideas about what is correct − that the world, for example, was created in seven days or that metaphysics is a lot of self-indulgent, unscientific foolishness, or that a person cannot alter her health by her intent − are unable to see through the paradoxes of life. They have assumed heavily defended, premature commitments to reality.

Again, paradoxes are windows to wisdom. Intellectual openings through which we may behold a vaster truth. Niels Bohr has been quoted as stating that no concept can be considered a great truth unless it gives rise to a paradox. The best way to approach a paradox or an issue in which we are presented with an either/or situation is to take a neutral stance, as I indicated in Chapter 2. Refusing to accept either position at the outset gives one the opportunity to examine both sides of an issue dispassionately. Often, each position holds an element of truth, and through neutrality we'll come to where the value lies. This process is not to be confused with failing to make up one's mind. It is just a more effective handling of paradoxes to realize that it is not always necessary to choose one truth over the other. Sometimes, it's better to award both positions their value.

To enjoy the fruits of the eclectic approach to health, it is not essential to have a complete grasp of the metaphysical nature of humankind and the Universe. Human consciousnesses apprehend concepts and ideas at different levels of comprehension, each according to its interests, abilities, and level of development. You do not have to understand the principles of internal combustion and bridge design and construction before you drive to the other side of the river. You are aware that certain principles of engineering were used and you accept the fact that the manufacturers of your car and the people who constructed the bridge understood and utilized them in the process. To believe in the existence of those principles and to trust them is essential, but it is unnecessary for you to understand what they are in order for you to own a car and risk making the trip.

Returning to the metaphor of the garden window in the blank wall, let us assume that the living room represents the commonly perceived reality of the Universe and humankind. It is undeniably real. But it is not the only real and valid way of perceiving ourselves and the Universe. What I hope to do is take you through the window into the garden, to another truth. The reality of the garden is not necessarily the only reality, any more than was the living room, but it is a different one. A truth is not necessarily the only truth. Again, we must avoid becoming rigidly committed to any one reality, even our old accepted one, as absolute, for our perception depends entirely upon our frame of reference. *To enter the garden and appreciate another truth – another way of viewing health and illness – certain concepts must be assumed to be true.* And they are true, just as the beliefs you held while in the living room were true.

The first concept to embrace is that humankind is an inseparable part of the Universe. The Universe, and the Earth specifically, are not here for our amusement and profit. We are not here to exploit and ravage in the name of greed and a healthy bottom line on a financial sheet. We are, on the contrary, an integral part of the Universe, just as each single cell within our bodies is an inseparable part of us. Since we are part of the Universe, it is incumbent upon us to act as if we are, to cooperate with nature rather than behaving like a cancerous mass of cells destroying everything we touch.

Second, you must conceive that the Universe is a living, sentient being. The Universe is an infinitely vast field of intelligent consciousness. From the theological point of view, this means that the Universe and God are one and the same. God did not create the Universe. God *is* the Universe. The Universe is God. From the perspective of our biologic nature, and through the focus of our physical senses, we see the Universe with our eyes and the instruments we have developed as matter/energy. Yet everything, the Universe and all it contains, is intelligent consciousness. The consciousness is aware; it has memory, purpose, precognition, and the ability to communicate and create.

According to accepted convention, some of what we observe is considered to be alive, and some is thought to be nonliving. However, everything is intelligent consciousness, it is *all* alive. Furthermore, we perceive the consciousness as various forms of matter and energy because of our desire and intent for it to appear that way. This is an important principle to comprehend, for this information is essential to understanding the nature of humankind. Therefore, let me state it in another, slightly different way: Through the action of our collective intent we have chosen to perceive the consciousness (the Universe) as atoms and molecules and to align them in various configurations to suit our purposes.

In many ways, scientific discoveries bear this out. Geoffrey Chew stated this in his "bootstrap" theory in the mid-1960s. Chew, a subatomic physicist, has written that there are no particles of anything. No protons, no electrons, no atoms, only interacting fields of energy that assume whatever form the observer wishes. At some time long past, all biologic entities reached an agreement that the consciousness would be perceived as this matter/energy stuff with which we are all familiar. One of the things we learned from the subatomic physicists is that matter and energy are different forms of the same thing. In my book *Reincarnation: The View From Eternity,* I coined the term "mattergy" to encompass the matter/energy paradox. It is by our intent that we "arranged" the world in this fashion, and it is by our intent, coupled with the cooperative intent of mattergy, that it continues to hold its form. The Universe as we perceive it is peculiar to our unique organization of thought and perception. Humankind did not create the Universe, but we did create the specific way in which we envision it. Stated in slightly different words, *the Universe, and our bodies as part of it,* is *intelligent consciousness actualized by our intent.*

The consciousness is made up of countless, infinitely tiny bits, which have been called "consciousness-units." Quanta, atoms, and so forth are formed around millions of these consciousness-units, which are what give mattergy its properties of life. It doesn't matter whether the atoms are part of a wisp of breeze, a pebble, a flower, or a human being, for the atoms are all formed around millions of consciousness-units and possess properties of life. These properties are consciousness, awareness, memory, intent, communication, creativity and precognition. In this sense, it is absolutely correct to say that the air and rocks are alive. The consciousness-units that formed the atoms manifest these properties of life, and they are part of a living Universe.

The stored memory contained in the consciousness-units directs the formation of various cells into tissues and organs from the single fertilized ovum. These infinitely powerful points of consciousness are transferred from generation to generation, through the mechanism of chromosomes in the reproductive cells, to guarantee the knowledge of how to construct a body. Continuing to define life in these terms, genes are blueprints formed by untold numbers of consciousness-units.

The Universe is made up of consciousness-units that are organized in various ways, floating in a sea of passively alert, undifferentiated consciousness. This sea is composed of consciousness-units and might be compared to an infinitely large and pure ocean. The quanta forming the protons, electrons, and neutrons making up the atoms of hydrogen and oxygen in the water molecules might then represent the consciousness-units. From the water, countless structures might be constructed, organized by the consciousness-units just as the face of the extra-terrestrial was formed from the ocean water in the movie, *The Abyss*.

Since matter is the materialization of thought – organized by these consciousness-units – then the "reality" we know is, in every way, a shared dream brought into being by our collective intent. By our unified purpose, we organized the consciousness into the patterns with which we are familiar and which we encounter daily. Keep in mind that it is only because of our narrow focus of attention that we perceive mattery as such. It is this limited perception that so often gives us the impression that there is no more to the world than we can document with our five senses. Some always knew that we consist of far more than the flesh-and-blood structures with which we are so familiar, and with which the average doctor deals when approaching our medical problems.

The living Universe, and we as living bits of that Universe, is far more complex than I have presented here. But it is only necessary here to comprehend that everything we know, and ever can know, is related to everything else. The Universe is nothing more than intelligent consciousness arranged in wondrous ways, with each element in contact and interrelating with all other elements. This applies to every quantum and atom, regardless of its location, in a grain of sand or in the most complex biologic entity that exists – a human being.

There's another way of looking at this broader reality as we move toward preserving our personal health: Everything that exists and occupies the world we know, and in which we interact, exists first in the *psychological* realm of the Universe. Since the Universe is conscious intelligence and we create our environment through our intent, everything must originally exist at a spiritual or psychological level before it is actualized in what we consider to be our temporal reality. This adds meaning to the statement that the reality we know and experience is a shared dream.

It is relevant that the Australian aborigines believe just that. They consider this "reality" in which we all live to be a dream and the dimension to which we go upon death as the true reality. Some aborigines who are psychically advanced individuals have the ability to "step out of their dream into reality." In doing so, it is reported, some can literally vanish from this earthly dimension, disappearing at will and reappearing wherever and whenever they like. In much the same way, Carlos Castaneda indicates that his teacher, Don Juan Matus, was able to "shift his assemblage point" and step into another reality while disappearing from this one. In fact, Castaneda reports that in his "final exam" as a sorcerer, he jumped off a cliff. He did not land in a broken heap on the rocks below because he had shifted his assemblage point and walked off into another dimension where the cliff did not exist.

This psychological framework, the true reality of the Universe, was discussed in Plato's *Republic*. Plato believed that the idea – the absolute concept of form – was the only reality, and that all else was an attempt to copy that idealized concept. This psychological reality has been called Framework II, the psychological dimension that contains all the ideas, thoughts, myths, fantasies, dreams, and concepts of every person who has ever lived or ever will live in the Universe. This psychological reality was what Jung was talking about when he spoke of the collective unconscious, and what Hindus call the Akashic records. But Jung's concepts, as he presented them, barely touched upon the vastness of all that is contained within Framework II. The concept of the Akashic records may come closer to the meaning.

Everything that exists is originally formed as a concept in Framework II as a belief, an idea, a contemplated action, a projected physical construct, or a philosophical thought. Everything in our everyday reality, which can be thought of as Framework I, has its origins in Framework II. Before the first table, computer, spoon, automobile, or rocket was ever built, it had to take form as a thought, constructed at the level of Framework II. As it was built, it became actualized in our "real" world of Framework I. In short, everything in Framework I is little more than a physical representation of the probabilities of Framework II. Framework II contains all the existing probabilities of being, and probabilities of probabilities....

Let's take a look at what this implies in our daily lives. When you get into your automobile to drive to the grocery store, the multitude of events that could happen exists all at once in Framework II. You could decide instead to drive to the post office, run your car off a bridge, drive across the country to see your aunt, or get out of your car and go back in the house for a nap. The possibilities are endless. Now, each of those things that you could do actually exists in the reality that is Framework II, and each is as real as the one you decide to actualize. By electing to drive to the store, you make that trip part of your reality in Framework I. It also becomes a reality for the grocer and everyone you meet along the way. Again, and this is important, *all the things you could have done are as real and valid as the one you chose to actualize.* Moreover, they are all *still* a part of Framework II and will remain there forever, to be acted upon whenever you like.

If you are exposed to a potent toxin, all the various probabilities exist at once in Framework II. You might not become ill. There is the probability that you will get sick but will have only a mild illness. There is also the probability of a severe illness. The probability exists that you might die. The crux of it all is that, to an extent so great as to be very nearly absolute, *you are free to choose, and do,* from the multitude of probabilities attended by your exposure to the toxin. And just as you are free to choose, you are to some degree free to change your mind and to actualize a different probability if you are dissatisfied with your first choice. Altering your course is not quite as easy as selecting the original one, but it can be effected and is achieved all the time.

This relationship between our ability to exercise intent in the creation of our temporal existence by choosing probabilities from Framework II has a very real effect on every aspect of our lives, including our health. We tend to make choices based upon internalized beliefs concerning our fate and destinies. Through the process of examining your belief structure, you can discover what your core beliefs are. If, for example, you adopted a hidden assumption that you will develop cancer as did your mother or father, it is perfectly possible for you to alter the future by dropping that belief and actualizing another probability lying in Framework II that does not see you dying that way. In every instant of your life you are selecting probabilities to actualize from Framework II. In every aspect of your being and at every moment of your life you have the option to choose a different probability.

Of course, this assumes that your early death from cancer is not part of a larger life plan. At times, certain things are beyond our control and ability to manipulate. If you find yourself dying despite your every attempt to address your core beliefs and your focused intent to recover, it is important that you not feel you have failed or that you are being punished. You must comprehend that at the level of Framework II you have agreed subconsciously to a different plan than the one you are knowledgeable of at a conscious level.

As you see, in the model for health and disease the aforementioned concept plays a vital role. It will be discussed later, but I want to make a point now while the concept of intent is fresh in your mind: ***Thoughts are things***. Every formulated thought is a "real something" that exists eternally in Framework II.

Physicists talk of infinite probabilities as the "sum over histories." They have mathematical symbols and equations to express the concept, but it works something like this. If a particle moves from its starting point at A and goes to point B, the sum over histories concept states that the particle had an infinite number of probabilities as to where it could travel – the same as when you got in the car to go to the grocery store. Physicists try to construct mathematical equations to explain why the particle arrived at B and did not go flying off in some other direction. But quantum mechanics has shown that, to some extent, the particle has the consciousness and the freedom and the intent that allow for its joyful cooperation. For this reason, it is entirely possible that it arrives at point B for no other reason than to please the physicist.

Subatomic physicists have frequently observed and commented on these actions of cooperative intent in their longstanding search for the basic building block of matter. When they tried to determine the nature of electrons, it was discovered that the electron's form depended upon the way the experiment was set up to observe it. If the physicist designed the experiment to view the electron as a particle, that was the way it appeared. If the experiment was devised to see the electron as a wave of energy, it appeared as a wave of energy.

The intent of the physicist determined the basic nature of the electron. Viewed from the standpoint of the electron, it was cooperating with the wishes of the physicist.

Recently, *Newsweek* magazine published an article describing the work of physicists at the University of Munich and the University of Maryland, who are now wrestling with the fact that photons in a particular experiment seem to know what the physicists expect them to do, even before the experiment is done, and that they behave accordingly! We are living in an intelligent, interactive, cooperative Universe in which we must come to grips with the evidence demonstrating that even photons and atoms are aware, communicate, and make choices.

When he stated that there are no particles of anything, Geoffrey Chew was right. You will remember he concluded that the Universe is made of interacting fields of consciousness that align themselves according to the wishes of the observer. Niels Bohr expressed the same thing when he said, "Isolated material particles are abstractions, their properties being definable and observable only through their interaction with other systems." That is exactly what the philosophers and metaphysicists have said for ages.

In some very real sense, the Universe is a conscious entity and we are, certainly, part of it as a living being. Because of our intense focus, we are more or less prevented from viewing the Universe in any other way than as the physical world we see. After all, we wanted to participate in this form of reality or we would not have created it in this fashion. But, clearly, what we see may not be all there is. And a good many among us are beginning to demonstrate that these other dimensions and perceptions are as real and valid as the one with which we are all familiar. Our way of perceiving the Universe should not be an excuse for denying the existence of other possibilities. If you are content remaining in your living room looking at the fly specks on the windowpane, do not deny others the reward of going into the garden. The view with which we are all familiar is, no doubt, a correct view of the Universe, but it may not be the *only* correct view. A concept may be true without being a solitary truth. Remember the discussion of the false notion that to accept one position we must reject all others.

On the basis of this brief and superficial introduction to metaphysics as it applies to medicine, one should appreciate the folly that the medical profession has allowed itself to perpetuate. It is patently clear that the multidimensional reality of our being far exceeds the mechanistic, "scientific" view that the medical profession adheres to so tenaciously. It is self-evident that a drastic opening of our basic beliefs is essential. To be a true healer and a physician of worth, a doctor must relinquish the idea that the old flesh-and-blood construct of the body represents a complete understanding. For a person to assume the role of physician and adhere to the limited view of humankind that is prevalent today is unworthy of the trust and confidence the public has placed in the profession. It is incumbent upon physicians to adopt a wider view of humankind and the Universe.

I am well aware that many of the things I have been writing about cannot be proven by a scientific method. No less do I understand that creative minds can come up with all sorts of reasons to refute metaphysical and psychological assertions. But many things we know to be true cannot be documented by any scientific means. You cannot prove that you love your spouse or your children. You might treat them kindly without actually loving them. If you do love them, how much? Is your love measured in pounds, inches, or watts? Science cannot answer all questions.

It is interesting that in a court of law a witness can testify to what she observed and heard. She is not required or expected to offer *scientific* proof that what she witnessed actually happened. If she testifies that she saw a man standing next to her draw a gun and shoot another, generally she is believed by the court, and the defendant can go to prison or to the electric chair on the basis of her statement alone. We seem willing to accept her observations in court concerning a crime, but if she were to say she saw a UFO or witnessed a psychic healing she would usually be disbelieved *because* she has no scientific proof.

I believe it is obvious that comprehending some different views of the Universe is critical to accepting a new model for disease. It is only upon accepting other truths that we can open our minds to vaster opportunities of learning and being. Admittedly, the implications go far beyond your getting over a bout of flu, healing your cancer, avoiding a heart attack, or maintaining your health. A broader view of our nature and our interaction with the rest of the Universe is essential to our experience as complete human beings.

CHAPTER FIVE

HEALTH OR ILLNESS

W E HUMAN BEINGS are remarkably more complex than we believe ourselves to be. Our physical senses give us such a limited view of ourselves. We are flesh and blood when viewed from the perspective of our biologic form; as we have learned, however, that is but one narrow view of our multidimensional being and only one pattern of perception. To deny the other dimensions to which I have referred is to deny our own vastness as a creation. Fully to comprehend ourselves, our health, our reasons for illness, and the mechanisms by which we recover, we need to expand our concept of humankind and accept our multidimensional self, as well as the multidimensionality of the Universe of which we are a part. This expansion is critical, for the distorted view of men and women as mechanical "things" has led to the intellectual box canyon in which the medical profession has taken refuge.

Since intent is the defining force in the Universe, then the human body is actually – and absolutely – a construction of thought. It is in a dynamic stage of constant formation and restructuring from the moment of its conception to the day it dies. Many biologists and researchers have told us that every year 98 percent of the atoms in our bodies are replaced, and that every seven years we have a totally new body, right down to the last atom. We take in millions of atoms of oxygen, which are incorporated into our tissues, with every breath, and we breathe out millions of molecules of carbon dioxide and water. The atoms in the food we eat replace other atoms throughout the body, which are then eliminated from the body as waste. The restructuring is constant. Half of your heart muscle is replaced every two weeks. Millions of blood and skin cells are destroyed every minute, and others are formed to take their place. This is accomplished through the creative intelligence, memory, and intent of the consciousness-units that are responsible for the formation of those cells and molecules.

The consciousness of every tiny portion of the Universe is infinite, infinitely complex, and infinitely interwoven. Every atom and every cell composing your body has within it an awareness of where it is and its function within the tissue of which it is a part.

From the practical point of view, all this means that your cells are intelligent, aware, individual units of living stuff. As individuated, living entities, each has multiple probabilities of action and behavior from which to choose, within the limitations of their being, just as you do when you get into your automobile to drive to the grocery store. And, given their abilities to differentiate purpose – to specialize their work within the complete organization of the body – it would seem clear that they are broadly free and that they enjoy the intent of cooperation. Cells cooperate with the intent of the tissues and organs within the total human body. Your cells, tissues, and organs follow instructions that are basic to all parts of the Universe. Those instructions have a dual purpose directed toward the best interests and purposes of the total organism, as well as toward the total goodwill of the Universe. All cells in a living body – muscle, bone, nerve, liver, kidney, connective tissue, and so forth – know what to do. If left alone, they have the ability to maintain themselves, to form new cells when needed, and to heal ills and injuries when they occur. This knowledge is maintained in the memory of the millions of consciousness-units of which the cells are formed. When a cell dies, the consciousness-units – like your soul – live on. They remain in place to organize a new cell where the old one was.

In addition to the basic instructions, each cell in your body responds to directions received from your conscious mind according to the belief system you have adopted. If you are totally convinced there is something wrong with your heart or liver, those cells will very likely alter their function to comply with your belief and produce the illness you have in mind. *This idea lies at the heart of selfhealing and at the opposite end of the process in which we produce disease through our internal beliefs.* Studies have been done on patients whose broken bones have failed to heal. Delving into their subconscious thoughts about their fractures revealed that, for various reasons, none of the patients thought their bones would heal properly. Other studies have been performed on individuals who have sustained a minor injury to an extremity, but whose entire extremity became disproportionately painful and nonfunctioning. This condition is known as reflex neuromuscular dystrophy or by the old term "causalgia." All of the causalgia patients in the study believed that their injuries were worse than the doctor had indicated. They were convinced that something was basically wrong with their limbs and that they would never be of any use again. Others, upon experiencing the pain of the original injury, react to the subconscious memory of an injury in another incarnation in which the injury to that body did not heal. This memory affects the behavior of the present body to continue the cycle of pain and disability.

In situations such as these, and in many others, cells do not see their actions as being "bad" or harmful. They see them as being cooperative and fulfilling the desires of a vaster organization of consciousness. One reason we become ill and grow older is that we see others around us doing those things and we do not question the pattern. As years pass, we anticipate becoming wrinkled, gray, and stiff, walking more slowly, growing forgetful, and taking on all those other characteristics usually associated with human aging. The bioconsciousness complies with that core belief and brings about the changes according to our instructions. This is not to deny the effects of free radicals and other pathologic events held to be at the heart of the aging process. It is only to say that both intent and physical events play parts in the process.

Humans are the focus of the doctor's professional efforts. It is our illnesses and injuries that he has been trained to diagnose and treat. To expand the scope of his vision and approach diseases from a perhaps more metaphysical frame of reference, he will need a concept of humankind different from the so-called scientific one he holds today. Following the Cartesian concept that body and mind are separate and distinct, physicians have busied themselves with superficialities, looking for physical mechanisms of one sort or another to fiddle with and adjust. Spiritual and metaphysical concepts and their relationship to illness and health have generally been rejected out of hand. This must change, for it is precisely these views that will open windows of opportunity that at present are carefully closed and bolted shut – defended by the official allopathic view of man, health, and disease.

We have said that all biologic creatures are spiritual entities that have, to a very real extent, *created* a body of one sort or another in order to exist in a biological setting. And I am convinced that within those bodies we are intended to enjoy life and learn from it. Being alive as a body of flesh and blood is meant to be experienced in its fullness. Humankind is meant to love, laugh, cry, play, and encounter the full gamut of emotional possibilities. Life is not meant to be all seriousness and hardship, filled with guilt and remorse, as most religions would have us believe. Life is a playing field upon which to learn. And that field can be whatever we choose to make it. One of my favorite quotes is from Oscar Wilde: "Life is too important to be taken seriously."

It is quite possible that human consciousnesses need a number of incarnations in order to assimilate the knowledge available from this framework of learning. Some souls may come only for specific bits of knowledge; others might need or want a more complete encounter. It is helpful to remember that each of us is but a splinter of a greater self. Emerson used the term "oversoul" to express the vastness of the overall spirituality of the Universe and us as part of that vast spiritual network. I use the term to indicate an individuated human consciousness and its multitude of interactions and relationships. When we are born, an extension of this oversoul invests itself into a specific existence, and as each physical body dies, the spiritual extension returns to the oversoul.

Certainly, during the life that takes shape between birth and death, many events happen to us. These events include the whole of life experience, from being fired from your job to falling in love, winning a game, and becoming ill or injured. But the mind always seeks to relate these events into a meaningful and instructive totality of experience. If I fall and mash my nose, at some level I automatically compare the injury with all others I have had of a similar nature. If I have a history of recovering quickly from smashed noses, my past experiences and intent will play a great part in how I react emotionally to the injury and in the rapidity of my recovery.

Similarly, untoward results in the past have the potential of interfering with present illnesses or injuries. In the opening chapter, the example of Bill's heel spur is a perfect one to illustrate these connections. In this example, the previous injury happened to occur in another life. Problems are raised when standard methods of therapy are applied without taking into account various metaphysical principles that may be contributing to the event. As in Bill's case, the average doctor does not understand and therefore completely misdiagnoses and mistreats such injuries. I know of no medical school in which even the mere possibility of a mechanism such as that in Bill's case is ever suggested, much less taught. Still, every physician has in his practice numerous patients suffering from diseases or symptoms caused or triggered by mechanisms outside the doctor's understanding. Invariably, the causes go undiscovered and often treatment fails, leaving the patients to endure lives of disability and pain. Not knowing the mechanisms that bring these conditions about, much less how to handle them, is hardly excusable for today's physician. There are far too many reports and examples for the thinking doctor to ignore. Once a doctor asked how come I knew these things. I replied, "How come you do not?"

Every doctor, indeed every person, has seen or heard of apparently meaningless and untimely deaths. At other times, people walk away from accidents that look as though they would have been fatal. These events are all, to one degree or another, the results of the intent of those involved. To give a few examples: some years ago, a young man driving in the Colorado mountains stopped at a scenic overlook and got out of his car for a better view. On the road a mile or two above him, a truck lost a wheel. The wheel came bouncing down the side of the mountain, struck the man in the head, and killed him before bounding off into the abyss. Was that a fluke of bad luck, was God playing a sadistic trick, or was it planned? Recently in Denver, a man was riding a motorcycle on Interstate 70. As he rode under an overpass, a dog fell off the overpass, knocking him from the bike and killing him, and the dog walked away unhurt. Another man, an elevator operator, was on the tenth floor of a building where he had left his elevator to go to the washroom. He returned to the bank of elevators and opened the door to what he erroneously assumed was his elevator. Without looking, he stepped into the open shaft and fell all ten floors, landing on the machinery below. Another man who had been waiting for an elevator stepped into the shaft immediately behind him and fell, landing on top of the elevator operator. The elevator operator's only injury was a sprained wrist and a couple of scratches. The other man was killed, his body badly broken and his skull split apart. We hear such stories at various times, shake our heads in wonder, and forget about them. Their explanations lie within the infinite probabilities of Framework II and in our understanding of the principles that operate along the lines of our personal intentions.

It often seems that each life is experienced for specific instructional purposes. Human existence seems set on teaching us lessons, such as how to handle wealth, poverty, good looks, fame, ill fortune, grief, or homeliness. Your life may also teach you about compassion, the bitter fruits of greed, impatience, or hate. It may teach you about love, boredom, and the importance of having fun, and it will certainly provide you with endless emotions and experiences that can only be appreciated from the circumstances of a biologic entity. One individual may plan a long life in order to experience the trials and difficulties of old age. Another may only desire to live to midlife and learn from illnesses or accidents. Behind the scenes, as it were, at the level of Framework II, arrangements are made that will best afford the opportunity to actualize the individual's intent and purposes.

Sometimes, there are focal points in life where the decision that is made will determine which line of probability will be followed. As conditions change, medical care improves, and life expectancy gradually lengthens, the life plans are adjusted to take those earthly conditions into the calculations. I believe that in some way, we choose these opportunities for our best potential of growth and wisdom and that we can, with deep reflection, change our minds and thus our experiences. If so, then we must come to understand and accept that we do not enter life merely to be beautiful and slim, not get wrinkles, to be wealthy happy, and to die in our sleep of old age. As a spirit within a body, we need to view the body as a vehicle in which we travel through the learning process. Since we are so intensely focused upon our physical being and do, indeed, think of ourselves as physical entities rather than spiritual ones, it seems clear that the spirit uses the body as an agent to discover many things about interactions with other human consciousnesses and about ourselves. Becoming ill can teach us to be compassionate toward others who are ill. A physical deformity can teach patience. Illness serves as an opportunity to observe how we cure ourselves and again to access our life's goals. In this way, we come to appreciate that *we are not our bodies.* Whether the illness is sought or accepted, once it happens, all these learning experiences can be had.

From this viewpoint, death that occurs early in life is not a mistake or tragedy. In fact, this is true of all deaths. Death is a new beginning. It gives the individual an opportunity to start another existence. Of course, rarely does anyone consciously choose to die. Focused as we are on our biologic nature, we find it hard to comprehend that, in many ways, our real existence lies in Framework II and beyond. It is here that the soul appreciates the lessons and wisdom that may come from what outwardly appear to be unfortunate events. It is at the level of Framework II that a person may choose or accept the purposes behind death and illness. In Framework II, concepts of guilt, the need for atonement, and condemnation do not exist.

Motives of guilt, condemnation, and damnation all block one's conscious perception of the meaning of death. If we resist death through fear, we lose the opportunity of free choice by blocking the energy flow that allows us to exercise the probability shift and choose life or joyfully accept the probability of death. Some, in contrast, choose potentially fatal situations as an opportunity to learn these things. In short, nobody dies an untimely death from any cause – by mistake, error, accident, or disease. Death offers an opportunity to proceed to new avenues of instruction and learning. Once individuals accomplish whatever they came for (or through inappropriate life choices ensure that they will never accomplish their purpose), death is the only way out.

I knew of a boy who was a senior in high school when he was diagnosed as having an osteogenic sarcoma of his thigh bone. He dated my granddaughter and took her to their senior prom – on crutches. He refused any treatment, saying that it was all right to die. He accepted the fatality of his situation. He had several long talks with my granddaughter, explaining that death is not a bad thing and that she should not worry about him or the fact that he had cancer. He died about a year later, having used his own passing to teach others how to approach and accept death.. He was closely attuned to the workings of Framework II and understood the purpose behind his death.

Some years ago, a person I knew went to a lake for his summer vacation. He didn't particularly like swimming but went along with his family because they enjoyed it. That year, he learned to water-ski and, I understand, was having great fun. The day before they were due to start for home, while he was water-skiing, he was struck by lightning and killed, literally out of the blue. There was no storm in the area and hardly a cloud, but at the age of thirty-four he was dead, killed by lightning. Ralph Warner did a psychic reading on the event and told me the lightning bolt had been produced for the singular purpose of freeing the man for his next incarnation. In any case, the fatal event certainly led his family toward a greater self-reliance. Understanding that these events are worked out in Framework II and referring to incarnational scenarios can expand our comprehension of our own lives at the working level. These case histories are examples of healing experiences that play both directions. If we do not understand death, we cannot comprehend life. If we do not understand illness, we cannot comprehend health.

Life events are not often predestined. On the contrary, every soul is free to choose: to follow the apparent plan or to reject it. Choices include the healing of illness, the avoidance of accident, or the shifting of probabilities. Everyone is free to be stubborn and free to act stupidly. In one sense, an individual has the option to thumb his nose at the gods and follow whatever course of action is dictated by that choice. As I said before, the built-in design of the Universe is based upon mutual support for all living creatures. This cannot be said strongly or forcefully enough: ***The cosmic intention is for us to live our lives in joyful cooperation and love for all of humankind and the totality of the Universe.***

The mind is a function of the spirit, not of the brain. When incarnation occurs, the mind fuses with the brain and nervous system and uses this organ system to communicate with the body and with other entities in the environment. The function of the mind that deals with events outside the body is known as the ego. Because of the intense interaction with things and events in the external environment, the ego seems to be separate from the rest of the mind, but it is not. It is wholly connected to another aspect of the mind that might be called the internal ego. This aspect deals with the bio-consciousness and with the knowledge and activities contained in Framework II. In a way, the conscious mind acts as an intermediary between these two egos and deals with everyday problems and events. The so-called subconscious mind is actually the part of the conscious mind where facts and memories that are not immediately required are stored. It's a basement of sorts, containing all the files of past events, impressions, and learned facts.

We have been taught that the subconscious is unfathomable, that it cannot be reached or understood without help from some individual who is trained to deal with those secret goings-on. But this is far from true. We simply have to learn to search within ourselves. And we are perfectly capable of doing this on our own. The subconscious mind is not the repository for unclean thoughts and horrible repressed memories, as Freud led us to believe. Delving into the subconscious is neither threatening nor dangerous. Keep in mind that the psychiatric profession has chosen to ignore the fact that Freud was both a cocaine addict and a pedophile.

It seems clear that during deep meditation and hypnosis the subconscious interacts with and receives the knowledge contained in Framework II, unaffected by the ego. The same process of information interchange takes place during sleep. It is here that the core beliefs set the tone of our being. And it is here that we can sort them out and choose other routes if we so desire. Looking into our subconscious beliefs is essential in the healing process. It is at this level that we can consciously begin to reinstruct our beliefs and our bio-consciousness to begin the healing process. We must include both, for if the belief structure is not addressed, instructing the bio-consciousness is often ineffective.

If you have adopted the core belief that you are sickly and will fall prey to every germ that comes along, it is very likely that this will happen. Possibly, you were a premature infant and were told that you were, therefore, subject to infections. This is a common statement made by doctors, and the parents of the premature child will usually pass this information along. While it is certainly true that during the first few weeks of life the premature infant has less resistance to infections, the condition does not persist into childhood unless we will it so.

Many people subscribe to the old wives' tale that sitting in a draft will cause a cold – so colds result.

Perhaps your mother was obese and told you that you took after her. To you this meant being fat, so you programmed your body and your metabolism to become obese as well.

Ominous and foreboding statements such as these tend to program the subconscious mind to accept many ideas concerning your body and your inability to fend for yourself. Your bio-consciousness takes these remarks as truths to be acted upon. These ill-conceived subconscious beliefs instruct your cellular consciousness in many ways. Perhaps it is not that you seek illness so much as that you feel totally powerless to do anything about it. In either case, you allow the illnesses to occur unchallenged.

If any of these scenarios fits your life experience, then to alter the cycle of illness, you must think back to the earliest times, when you first arrived at these beliefs. Regardless of the loving intent of those who implanted the false ideas, they were wrong, and you must come to believe this without question. This is called reinstructing your autonomous reflex system. Since you, no doubt, heard these things countless times, or had them implied to you in many ways, it will be necessary to talk to yourself numerous times before your bio-consciousness begins to believe that you are free of your false instructions. Meanwhile, you need to speak to your bio-consciousness – using "we" – and redirect it. Your body must be told that it remembers its original prime directive to remain healthy and resist infections and illnesses. It must be told to start acting upon that principle, following its original genetic plan, rather than upon the misguided statements of others. Again, it may take many instructions over an extended time to accomplish the task – a minimum of once daily over a three-week period. But it will work, for the body and its physiologic behavior is almost exclusively a thought construction.

Illness and health are direct expressions of the spirit, its desires and intentions, set within the internal plan of the person and the society of which he or she is a member. *If left alone, the body is perfectly capable of keeping itself healthy.* It is also constantly attuned to instructions from the internal ego. Our bodies continuously interact with bacteria, viruses, yeasts, mites, and fungi, many of which live within or on us in perfect harmony. They are there, ready and waiting to produce an illness at appropriate times, if that is our desire. Once you have "suffered" enough, and because it is not within your belief system that you will die of a minor illness, your body's defenses come to your "rescue" and you recover.

Not long ago, I happened to witness an incident between a woman and her two-year-old child. A minor accident occurred in which the child was bumped in the mouth and sustained a tiny cut on the inside of his lip. I looked at the cut and saw that it was of no importance, just a little blood and a slight amount of discomfort for the child. Nonetheless, the child's mother almost became hysterical over the event. She was obviously in a panic and, of course, the child reflected his mother's anxiety. Some time later I learned that he had sustained several injuries of like severity, and that in each instance the mother had rushed him to the emergency room of the local hospital to be "treated" by a doctor. The woman's actions served as a powerful, instructive lesson for the child. First, he was being taught that every tiny injury is a frightening event. Second, he was learning that his mother was totally incapable of handling any sort of crisis, regardless of how minor it might be. Third, he was being instructed that he must run to the doctor for every small pain or scratch. Last, and not least, he was learning not to evaluate a situation himself, but to run to some figure of authority every time something goes wrong. I can see him as a grown man, dashing to the doctor's office to be assured that his cold is not going to turn into pneumonia, or that he is not going to die of blood poisoning from the scratch on his finger. By means of his childhood experiences, he will have learned to be fearful and to create disasters from insignificant events. Unfortunately, his body consciousness will gladly comply with this belief system.

On the other hand, the child who does not hear these things or, in his innate wisdom, chooses to ignore them, is apt to think of himself as strong and healthy. He will have complete confidence that his body can take care of itself. Rarely will he get a cold or the flu and, if he does, it will probably be the result of his body defenses being diminished due to some stressful situation, or the body's need to exercise its defense mechanisms. In any case, it most likely will be both mild and of short duration.

Illnesses other than infections may also be programmed by the core beliefs of individuals. Heart attacks, cancers, ulcers, and every other illness imaginable are sometimes the result of an unconscious desire to be ill for some reason, or ignorance of the fact that being well is an option. In these situations, the bio-consciousness either chooses a common illness or allows a disease that started spontaneously to go unchecked. Probably every person reading this book has had several cancers develop that now lie dormant or have already been eliminated by the body's defenses. The only one that will ever be diagnosed will be the one that your body allows to remain unchecked because, at some level and for some specific reason, you have wished or allowed it to develop. Why would anyone choose to have a cancer? To understand this question, we must come to grips with a new concept of disease: the principle that diseases and injuries are wake-up calls to re-examine our lives.

Cancer represents new growth in more ways than one. First, it offers a person a way out of this life. It is socially acceptable to die of cancer, whereas suicide is frowned upon. But why not an accident or a heart attack that could be relatively painless and quick? The answer may lie in the individual's needing a protracted death as a learning experience. Perhaps she chooses it because she realizes that her family needs to face certain aspects of life and death and that giving them some months to grapple with those issues will be helpful. Perhaps it is to ease her way out of their lives – to let them meet her departure with a certain relief rather than shock. Such a death may, in one way, be an act of love. These are valid reasons why the patient should always be given the diagnosis rather than keeping it a secret.

Many years ago, when I was practicing in Champaign, Illinois, I had a patient with a spot on his chest X-ray that appeared to be a cancer of the lung. The family told me in no uncertain terms that I was not to tell the man his diagnosis if it turned out to be malignant. I informed his wife and daughter that I had a moral and legal responsibility to give the patient his diagnosis. I attempted to explain that he was the person with the disease and the one who would have to deal with the consequences should it turn out to be cancer. They were adamant that he should not be told, saying that he would be unable to cope with the diagnosis and would commit suicide. I told them that if he decided to commit suicide, that was his choice. I doubted he would take such an action, but I intended to give him his diagnosis in any case.

After the surgery, when the diagnosis was confirmed, I told the man that he had lung cancer. His response was a huge sigh of relief. He said that knowing the truth, even though it was cancer, was better than the anxiety and uncertainty of not knowing the diagnosis. He asked how much time he had, and I told him that at least 70 percent of patients are dead in about a year. I spent a great deal of time talking with him. I explained that he was only going to die once and, until that day arrived, he was alive and should continue to live a full life. I helped him understand that life had always been an uncertain event, never knowing if the next moment would be his last. I jokingly added that with any luck he might fall down and break his neck or be killed in a car accident and not live to die of his lung cancer. In short, he did not know what the future held for him. As I anticipated he would, the patient took it very well. But his wife and daughter were very angry at my having told him the diagnosis. Not only did they refuse to speak with me, they insisted that he change doctors.

A year later, I read his obituary in the newspaper. Some months after his death, the daughter came to see me. She hugged me and apologized for all the hateful things she had said about me. She went on to say that her father's last year had been one of the best of their lives. He had helped his wife learn how to write checks and handle their family affairs. They had talked about life and death and what it all meant. They had discussed many things that neither his wife nor his daughter had any idea he even thought about, much less was concerned about. She went on to say that if her father had not been aware of his diagnosis, they would not have been able to have the visits they did. Perhaps, cancer is not always the horrible thing we are led to believe. In this case, it was a blessing that drew the family closer, even as it brought this life to its end and allowed a new one to begin.

Of course, I realize that by telling the man he had about a year to live, I was likely helping him schedule his death. His cells, no doubt, responded to the belief in "one more year" and programmed his death according to that timetable. Anyway, the calendar ran true to the prognosis.

In the same fashion, the woman who has a family history of breast cancer is very apt to produce a cancer according to her own and the doctor's expectations. If the particular woman has accepted as a core belief that it is her fate to die of cancer as did her mother, grandmother, and aunts, her cells will most likely joyfully cooperate. In order to comprehend this seemingly destructive process, you must recall that the bio-consciousness takes instruction from the vaster consciousness of the mind. Just as the molecules joyfully cooperate with the intent of the cells, the cells cooperate and acquiesce to the stated directions of the mind. This cooperation carries to the extent that the cells abandon their prime directive to reproduce normally and remain healthy, and set about producing the appropriate tumor or illness. Since this is true, then all of the self-administered breast examinations and mammograms can strongly reinforce a woman's core belief and may even assist in instructing her bio-consciousness to produce a cancer. Information concerning cancer and other diseases from which we "must defend ourselves" in order to avoid becoming "victims" may very well serve as a blueprint for illness.

Most physicians who see cancer running in families subscribe to the idea that it is hereditary. To a degree this appears to be true. We certainly know how to breed strains of mice that will cooperate and develop malignant tumors of the breast. So, undoubtedly, a tendency to develop cancer may be inherited. But whether any one individual within a "cancer family" develops a tumor is another thing. It may well be that internal instructions to the cells in the form of core beliefs are a necessary addition to whatever genetic factors may be present in order for cancer to develop. However, I know of no oncologist who has considered the possibility that families bring cancers on themselves by unwittingly teaching each other what to expect. It is feasible that self-examination for breast tumors, mammograms, and publication of the danger signals for cancer may actually increase the incidence of the disease by focusing the attention of the individual on that area of the body. Of course, each patient must define her own health care under the advice of her own doctor. But if she is fearful of developing breast cancer, it is possible that this constant attention may be taken by the bio-consciousness as an intent to produce one. This is not to say that an occasional checkup is harmful, but a monthly ritual performed by a frightened woman has the potential of producing the very cancer she fears.

Our society has developed a sort of "disease of the month" mentality. When I was in medical school, the most common cancer in men was stomach cancer. Then cancer of the lung became popular, and cancer of the stomach all but disappeared. Following this, we went through a period when everyone was talking about their emotional difficulties and the psychotherapy they were receiving. A few years ago, news articles began talking about colon cancer and people responded with an increase of colon tumors. Now that we have AIDS, nobody seems concerned about herpes. Another example is demonstrated by the recently developed blood test to detect cancer of the prostate gland. Men are now being urged in advertisements, public service announcements, talk shows, and by their doctors, to have the test performed. And they are responding in droves. I read recently that there has been a sudden increase of no less than 600 percent in the incidence of prostate cancer! The article went on to say that about half of the cases would not have been diagnosed were it not for the new test, but that still does not explain the 300 percent actual increase in the disease in the last few years.

What has happened may be something like this. A person who, at the psychological level, is wanting out of this life most likely chooses the cancer that comes most readily to mind. Perhaps he has already developed a small prostate cancer that would have remained dormant for many years, possibly all his life. But in their desire to comply with the man's unconscious wish, the cancer cells activate and begin to grow. In other instances, by focusing his attention on his prostate, he may actually instruct the cells to alter themselves, and in doing so, they become cancerous.

The interaction between the cellular consciousness, the internal ego, and the conscious mind is somewhat similar to the relationship of the sorcerer's apprentice with the broom. I'm sure you know the story in which the sorcerer's apprentice was assigned the task of filling a cistern with water from a well. Instead of doing it himself, he used a magic command to bring a broom to life and do the task for him. The problem arose when the cistern became full but the broom kept bringing more water until the place was flooded. The apprentice didn't know the command to cause the broom to halt its activity. It took the sorcerer to give the command to stop the broom.

If a commanding general gives his army orders to attack a particular objective, each soldier is made aware of the command to attack. As he accepts the assignment, each soldier goes about his business doing those things necessary to conduct the battle. The order to fight supersedes all other orders received previously concerning marching in parades, keeping the camp policed and clean, and other peaceful missions and activities. Time passes, and then a moment comes when the general decides to make peace and cease the attack. A truce is decided upon and the treaty papers are signed, but if the general doesn't bother handing down the order to cease fire, then the battle will continue. In such a scenario, divided purpose develops in which the general continues to talk about the peace he has negotiated while his army continues to fight the battle.

This is exactly what happens in many instances of illness and disease. The cells respond to certain core beliefs given to them by the internal ego that override their prime directive to repair themselves and maintain a state of health. Although the person may consciously wish to be well and may talk about licking his illness, the cells continue to behave according to what they feel are overriding directions to the contrary. To solve this conflict, we must look to our core beliefs and assumptions. If we have instructed our bodies to become ill or have unwittingly adopted a death wish, we need to address our bio-consciousness with different instructions, using the pronouns "we" and "us" in order to make certain that the cells understand we are talking to them.

In our culture, medicine and doctors sometimes act as unspoken messengers. In his book *The Doctor, His Patient and the Illness,* Dr. Michael Balint states that the most powerful therapeutic agent the doctor has at his command is his own personality. He has the capability of bringing about a cure in the patient by his will and intent. A charismatic doctor who loves his patients will invariably have better results treating diseases than the physician who remains reserved and aloof.

Often medicine or surgery works for the simple reason that the patient believes it will. As a result, the cells think, "Well, if you're serious enough to have an operation, then we'd best start getting better." This is why studies have shown that sham procedures are often remarkably effective. A sham operation is one in which the patient is told that a certain operation will be performed; then the surgeon makes an incision into the body, sews it up, and informs the patient that all went well. In controlled studies, the results of such procedures have often proven as dramatic as in patients on whom the real operation was performed. This same principle operates in the use of placebos. Approximately one-third of patients react as well to placebos as they do to real medicine. Most doctors view this phenomenon as evidence of the patients faking their problems, but it is far more likely that their bodies have responded to the intent of the patient to recover. What is not generally known is that another one-third of patients react in the opposite way. Regardless of how strong or effective the medicine may be, they report that it does not work at all.

In other cultures, other healing modalities are often just as effective as the ones we brag about. Dances, incantations, bells, sand paintings, crystals, and such serve the same purpose – that of focusing the intent upon getting well, and thereby obtaining the cooperation of the bio-consciousness. Health, illness, and our ultimate response to illness are products of our belief system and our spiritual intent.

Many diseases and conditions are caused by just the sort of thing we have been talking about, in which the bio-consciousness continues to act upon previously made assumptions. One such action is known as a conditioned reflex. When a conditioned reflex forms, something happens to the body at the same time that another event is taking place. The subconscious mind associates the two, and the internal ego instructs the cells to reproduce the same physical reaction every time a similar event occurs.

One of my patients injured his back when he was a child. His mother had been in the act of scolding him for climbing a tree when he fell from the tree and injured himself. She lectured him, saying that he would not have been hurt if he had not disobeyed and had used better judgment. In truth, the boy probably would not have fallen if his mother had not been yelling at him, but that's another story. The boy recovered from the injury and all was supposedly forgotten. But his bio-consciousness and his internal ego did not forget. As a result, the two totally unrelated events – the scolding and the injury – were linked in the boy's mind. As he grew older, he suffered from a bad back for which there seemed to be no pattern of occurrence. Sometimes his back pain appeared to result from work; at other times it would start when there had been no unusual activity. He had seen numerous doctors and orthopedic surgeons. One of them even diagnosed him as having a ruptured disc and performed surgery. But the surgery was of no help.

Having learned that I used hypnosis, he came to my office seeking relief from his back pain. Under hypnosis, he revealed the link between the scolding incident and his injury. The trigger for the episodes of pain was any confrontation in which he viewed himself as being guilty of an error or misjudgment. Thus, if his boss dressed him down for some slip in performance, or if he had an argument with his wife for which he felt in some way responsible, however slight or insignificant the episode might be, his cellular consciousness produced the pain and muscle spasm in the same fashion as in the original injury. While he was still under hypnosis, I called his attention to the events and let him see that they were connected only by having happened at the same time. The scolding had not directly caused his injury. After that session, the man had no more back trouble. By bringing his subconscious mind and his cellular consciousness to a greater understanding of the erroneous connection between the guilt of error and his pain, we were able to remove, instantly, a long-standing conditioned reflex. This sort of situation is almost exactly the same as what happened to Bill's heel in the first chapter of this book. In Bill's case, his internal ego was reminded of the other injury by a slight pain in his heel caused by standing on the ladder. In this last case, the cellular response was triggered by feeling guilty.

Just as common are the times when illness is actively sought. The hardworking individual who finds it difficult to take a day off can take a few days of rest if he has the flu, and no one will think less of him. He can't tell his boss that he is going home just to rest or to get away and go fishing. No doubt, the boss would not approve of such a thing. But several days of a legitimate illness serve much the same purpose. His internal ego is well aware of this and instructs his bio-consciousness accordingly. In response, his cellular consciousness gladly joins forces with a virus to supply him with the symptoms he needs. He is not malingering – he is really sick, with the fever, headache, cough, and muscular aches to prove it.

Studies have been done on men who had heart attacks. In virtually every instance, the studies revealed that these men had been subconsciously looking for rest or a way out of an untenable situation.

When I was in surgical training, it was standard practice to instruct patients who had undergone abdominal surgery not to return to work for six to eight weeks. Every patient, however fit, was expected to be weak and unable to work following such an operation. And so they all were cautioned not to lift, not to drive a car, not to go up and down stairs, and so on. After I learned that patients can hear even while they are under a general anesthetic, I started giving them suggestions while they were on the operating table. I would tell them how good they would feel now that their gallbladder had been removed or whatever the case was. I encouraged them to return to work immediately and to perform any physical activity they desired. I gave their bodies many instructions about being able to eat normally, eliminate wastes, and many other things. The upshot of this novel approach was that my patients left the hospital within one to four days following major surgery and most returned to their normal activities immediately. Nobody's wound fell apart. Nobody got an infection, had to be catheterized, or suffered gas pains. The truth was that the other surgeons' patients who received the standard spiel of instructions and warnings with a list of forbidden activities did exactly what their doctors suggested as well. The other doctors unwittingly programmed their patients to have pain, nausea, gas pains, and a long recovery time.

In every instance, whether we are dealing with illness or health or recovery from an illness, the keys to the outcome are desire and intent. It is readily seen that the desire may be at a completely unconscious level. Unfortunately, the medical profession as a whole is largely unaware of these dynamics of health and disease. Working on the principle that we are victims of illness that happens to us, doctors too often assume the stance of defenders of their patients. Their every action is to fight off the attack of some illness, germ, or virus. They see their patients as victims of cancer, heart disease, or gallstones when, more accurately, their patients have allowed or sometimes created illness in a sort of cosmic promenade of psychological and spiritual events.

Understand that *as long as we see ourselves as victims of illness dependent on the ministry of doctors, we need to be very careful if we decide to ignore that belief.* All healing systems are effective if the patient believes in their worth. It is the belief in the system and the intent to become well that determines whether a sick person will recover. The Navajo Indian who has the medicine man create a ritual sandpainting receives treatment just as effective as does the stockbroker in New York who goes to a super-specialist for the latest drug. If the stockbroker became ill while visiting the reservation and sought the help of the medicine man, it is highly unlikely that the treatment would be of much use, for the broker would not believe that such superstitious activity could be effective. At the same time, if the Navajo became ill in New York, he might be suspicious of a white man's drugs, and his belief system might lessen or completely counter the effectiveness of such measures. The Navajo might well need to return home and have his medicine man do a sandpainting in order to recover fully.

Incantations, dances, bells, poultices, faith healers, massage, copper bracelets, eagle feathers, and other forms of healing art can hasten recoveries *if they coincide with the belief structure and intent of the patient.* At best, any form of therapy is only an adjunct to the healing activities and abilities of the mind and the cellular consciousness.

One criticism of this line of thinking was brought to my attention by an acquaintance who posed an example of an individual with a heart attack. Let us take a theoretical man who suffers a massive coronary and is rushed to the hospital. There, the doctors attempt to stabilize him, find that the damage is very severe, and proclaim that he must have immediate surgery or he will die. He is taken to the operating room, where balloon angioplasty is attempted and fails. Immediately, coronary artery bypass surgery is performed on three vessels. The man makes a satisfactory recovery and goes home to live another two years.

This is a common scenario, acted out many times a day in hospitals across the country. However, we need to ask some hard questions about this chain of events. First, are we truly certain that the man would have died without the surgery? Who is to say with total authority? What if the grafts had clotted shut a week or two after he went home? They often do, so why did the man live two more years with the circulation to his heart no better than before he went to the hospital in the first place? What would have happened if the same man had been living in the backwoods of Alaska and no hospital had been available? Would he inevitably have died?

Remember that nobody dies at any time without at some level wishing to do so. The man obviously did not want to die or he would have done so, regardless of how aggressive or skilled the surgeon and the doctors might have been. On the other hand, since these modern surgical methods were available to him, he may have put his faith in them and believed that without them he would not survive. Had they been denied him or delayed, perhaps because he did not have insurance, he might have altered his probabilities and accepted death as inevitable or necessary, given the circumstances. Perhaps he would even have died in order to make a social statement that he had been unable to receive proper care for lack of insurance.

Had he been in the Alaskan wilderness, he would have been aware that coronary care units, surgery, and such were not a possibility. In that context, yielding to a massive heart attack would have been choosing to die, and so he might not have allowed it. Electrocardiograms often reveal the presence of old, healed heart attacks when the patient can give no history of ever being sick. In a study performed by a Harvard professor in Ukraine, electrocardiograms were performed on many healthy individuals who were over one hundred years old. A number of them showed evidence of past myocardial infarctions. On questioning, some recalled having had a period of chest pain when they were unable to work as hard as usual.

My point is that doctors do not know for certain who will live and who will die. That is not so strange when one considers that most of the time they don't know why the individual became ill in the first place. People die when they intend to die, and they become ill when they intend to be ill.

It should be patently evident that we are in control of our lives at all times. Nothing happens to us in which we are not in some way complicit – this includes illness, injury, and death. Our bodies are actually constructed according to our thoughts. They are being rebuilt constantly and renewed at a breakneck pace according to the wisdom of the cells themselves. Problems arise when our cellular consciousness receives instructions that override the primary intent of the cells to remain healthy. In these cases, the cells comply with the sometimes hidden commands in ways that are often detrimental to the physical body. To be healed, then, the ill must first reach inward and learn to be well again.

CHAPTER SIX

A BASIS FOR THE
NEW MODEL OF
DISEASE

I T'S TIME TO ACCEPT a more accurate paradigm for the development of illness. Clearly, we can no longer afford to ignore the flaws in the old models. In the preceding chapters, you've been introduced, directly and indirectly, to some new beliefs. At this point, I hope you agree that we must begin with a different concept of what constitutes a human being if we intend to expand health care beyond the technical exercise it is today.

We must abandon the belief that a human being is a body with a spirit that has little or no effect upon the body's well-being. On the contrary, as I've stated repeatedly, spirit, in a very real way, *creates* the body. We've learned that each human spirit, or consciousness, is a unique collection of untold trillions of consciousness-units that organize mattergy about them to form atoms and molecules. The wisdom and memory of the consciousness-units within the matter clearly direct the creation and organization of the genes, molecules, cells, and tissues that make up the body. The biological body is the physical representation of the spirit cast in flesh and blood.

When we perceive a person to be miserable and unhappy because of some chronic illness, we have our thinking backward. It is far more likely that he is chronically ill because he is a miserable and unhappy person. The state of his spiritual being is reflected in the body of his own construction. This is in direct contrast to the allopathic assertion that, more than anything else, we are each a product of our genes – that we inherit things such as obesity, heart attacks and cancer and are only victims of invading germs and abnormal physiology.

Of course, genetic inheritance is of great importance and does serve as the creative blueprint for the cells to follow, but it is *not* a blueprint chiseled in stone. Genes create *tendencies* or *potentials* to develop certain physical and mental characteristics, conditions, and diseases. At the same time, there is an interplay between the genetic plan and the social and emotional environment that surrounds the individual. Along with our physiological tendencies, we inherit a particular cellular sensitivity that makes the cells more or less likely to follow those tendencies.

This cellular sensitivity also provides the potential for curing ourselves should we find ourselves with a genetically induced illness. This is possible because the cellular receptivity is directed not only toward acting upon the genetic tendency, but also toward reacting to the instructions from the internal ego. There is potentially great danger in genetic tests that reveal the presence of certain genes associated with various diseases. The implication is that the patients are powerless victims of their own genetic makeup, and this belief is dangerous. By worrying about the results of such tests, uninstructed patients may greatly increase the chances of their worries coming true. On the other hand, if the patients can be led to use knowledge of their genetic tendencies as an opportunity to reinstruct their bioconsciousnesses, then they might well entirely offset their genetic codes.

Cancer (and all diseases, inherited or otherwise), will develop only if the person is not fulfilling his greatest constructive potential. In fact, it is spiritual conflict that causes illness to develop. Unresolved conflict with their mothers is a major factor in women who develop breast cancer. In other situations where there is a family history of breast cancer, a hidden assumption may be adopted by a young girl that cancer will be her fate as well. Acupuncturists have discovered alterations in the flow of energy in specific meridians months before a physical illness develops in the organ related to those meridians.

It seems clear that our lives are meant to teach us, that we live to gain in wisdom that can be attained from no other plane of being. In addition to learning the importance of being loving and forgiving, we must learn to handle the myriad problems of interpersonal relationships we have as biologic entities. The incarnational phase of learning may include situations that we see as undesirable, such as being crippled, ill, or mentally retarded. But can we not learn compassion for others by observing the disabled? Can we not learn from the crippled body of a loved one? Yes, but for some, personal experience is the best way. The endless possibilities of life scenarios themselves constitute our greatest challenges for spiritual learning.

It is equally clear that each of us has a certain finite time to accomplish these tasks. When that time has elapsed, the only way for a human consciousness to go on to other learning opportunities is for the spirit to leave the body. This is called death. Our society – and our physicians – must learn to accept that, in this context, death is never premature. We tend to accept the death of an older person who perhaps has weathered the ravages of cancer or some debilitating disease. On the other hand, when a child or an adult in his prime dies, we are appalled and wail at the unfairness of it all.

We must all, doctors and patients alike, come to grips with the reality that no one dies or becomes ill who does not, at some deeper level of being, choose to do so. Do not forget about that marvelous, labyrinthine system of spiritual interaction we have called Framework II in which all manner of creative associations and events are formulated with the total cooperation of every living soul in the Universe. In the context of "Framework II", no death or illness should be thought of as unorchestrated or inexplicable.

Because we are trained and conditioned to feel guilty about and place blame for every untoward event, however small or insignificant, it will be difficult, but let us strive to put that concept aside once and for all. It is vital that each of us accept full and complete responsibility for our own well-being. This means every aspect of our state of being. We must accept total responsibility for the condition of our lives, our happiness, our financial status, our social position, our relationship with others, our health, our illness, our injuries, and our recoveries or continued infirmities. By accepting personal accountability for our condition, we can no longer think of ourselves as victims of anything.

We cannot – must not – believe that we are victims of society, our parents, the boss, our race, a drunk driver, cancer, heart attacks, AIDS, disease germs, accidents, or anything else. Once we accept that we are not victims, but are each to a very great extent the authors of our situation, we empower ourselves to do something about it. After all, *if we created our plight, or were at least complicit in its development, then we are empowered to alter our circumstances*. The individual who sees herself as a hapless victim of society has a tendency to wallow in her problems rather than actively doing something about them. She may complain loudly about what happened to her and how society is to blame and what society should do to atone for its actions. The woman who sees herself as a victim of breast cancer, or the man who views himself as a victim of heart disease, searches further and further outside the self for help. As a victim, the patient must unceasingly seek a newer drug, or a hospital with better facilities, or a doctor with more certificates on his consultation room wall.

"Victims", by the very act of seeing themselves as victims, also view themselves as powerless – impotent in their plight. The individual who embraces the truth that he created his illness through his core beliefs or his stance in life – or who, because of those beliefs cooperated with the illness once it started – must also believe that he can create another condition. He is not to blame for his illness, nor should he blame someone else. He should instead ask himself what it is that he should learn of life, and then set about altering the circumstances and curing himself.

Accepting responsibility for your destiny empowers you to act on your own behalf.

These concepts are *critical* to comprehend. *We are here, in part, to learn these things and, if we do it well in a given life, perhaps we will not have to go through it again.* Illness, injury, and eventual death are essential to the biologic state. If we do not grasp the concept at this incarnate level, we will never progress beyond the point where guilt and fear orchestrate our lives.

As part of the living entity we call the Universe, we exist in a cooperative alliance with every other living thing. In addition to the plants and animals in our external environment, we share our bodies with millions of viruses, yeasts, fungi, bacteria, and other tiny organisms. It is a symbiotic relationship, for they serve many useful purposes the medical profession has yet to understand. The same viruses that cause disease may well serve as messengers or activators of normal body processes at other times. At those times when the spirit is seeking an illness, the bacteria and viruses may just as gladly cooperate.

As a biological entity living in this dimension, any individual may face occasions when she is overwhelmed with a large number of bacteria from without. Such things happen, for example, when one eats unrefrigerated chicken or potato salad in which salmonella or staphylococcus bacteria have managed to grow. Both types of bacteria have the ability to produce a severe gastrointestinal upset. Such a situation can serve to instruct us to keep food refrigerated. The enteritis itself might be of benefit to the body by serving to sharpen its defensive mechanisms. Others might have eaten the same potato salad and ingested the same amount of bacteria and toxin and have not become ill because they did not personally need a lesson, or perhaps because they can learn by observing others' illnesses. Other episodes of minor illness such as colds and flu no doubt perform the same sort of service.

In this sense, most accidents are not truly accidental. Ninety percent of all accidents are sustained by only 10 percent of the population. These "accident-prone" people are well known in the world of industry. Others who on occasion have a mishap have been shown in various surveys to have had something in their lives that made them seek an accident on that particular day. Repeated accidents are a bit like localized suicide, in which the person kills or injures small pieces of himself from time to time – a finger here, a toe there. Again, like an illness, an accident can be highly instructive, serving as a window of opportunity to evaluate one's life and to look at the direction one is going, perhaps simply to pay more attention to what one is doing.

I was still practicing medicine when this new model for disease was presented to me. My friend, the clinical psychologist Ralph Warner, spelled it out so clearly that I could not miss the truth. Ralph had just finished telling me that doctors never actually save lives.

"You mean I have never saved anyone's life – not even one?" I asked.

"No," he replied, smiling. "You doctors never understand."

"Well, then, what's the point of being a doctor?"

"Your purpose is to aid people who are sick and help them in their recovery, to relieve their pain and suffering, and then to use your skills to determine when death is inevitable. When that time comes, you should direct your efforts toward keeping your patient as comfortable as possible. But you should not interfere."

That concept is totally opposite to anything taught in medical schools. The entirety of medical training is directed toward diagnosing diseases, curing them, and preventing death. So I posed a medical situation for Ralph to address in light of what he had just told me. I outlined a hypothetical medical problem in which I fail to do Pap smears on a woman. Some years later she is found to have an invasive, far advanced carcinoma of the cervix. Following the discovery of the cancer and in spite of adequate radiation therapy, the patient dies of her disease within a fairly short time. I went on to explain that, if I had done yearly Pap smears, more than likely the cancer would have been diagnosed no later than Stage I, in which a cure is almost assured. In a situation such as I had outlined, would I not be responsible for the woman dying of cancer perhaps years before she ordinarily would have died?

Ralph's reply was that the woman would not die before her time, regardless of what I had done. He said that if I made the early diagnosis of the cancer and through treatment it was eliminated, she would simply have had to find some other method to leave this earthly plane. The fact that she died, signified that she was ready to do so. If I had cured the cancer, she would have had to arrange an accident, a stroke, or some other means of exiting this life. He explained that the Universe is very creative.

To prove his point, Ralph went on to state that no lives were saved when the speed limit on interstate highways was reduced to fifty-five miles per hour. Disbelieving, I got out a book containing death statistics in the United States and showed him the big drop in traffic fatalities during those years.

"Yes, that's true," he countered, "but look at the total deaths for those years." And he was right! The total number of deaths in the United States from all causes was unchanged!

Ralph went on, "The people who wanted to check out simply had to find another way to do it. When it is time for someone to die, he will die. If the medical profession makes it difficult to die of one disease, then the person simply chooses another way. People get sick when they want and die when they want, and not before."

I looked at the other causes of death listed in the report. Sure enough, during those years there was a slight increase in other deaths – a few more deaths due to pneumonia, diabetes, liver diseases, heart problems, other accidents, and so on. The total number of deaths from all causes in those years had remained unchanged. Gasoline consumption may have gone down, but not deaths.

Central to the new model of illness is that the patient is *never* a victim. At the very least, he participates by allowing the disease to develop. As I have said, this statement is not made in order to place blame on the patient, nor to shift responsibility, nor for the purpose of letting the medical profession off the hook. It is simply a more accurate model of the cause of disease. In the new paradigm, the patient is responsible not only for his illness but also for his recovery. The very most a patient should expect from his doctor is some help on occasion.

I know this concept will not be pleasing to doctors' egos, for they have been trained that it is their mission to cure people and save lives, rescuing patients from certain death. Many patients will also object, for it will require that they take responsibility for their own good health. Adopting a model for disease in which patients are responsible for their own illnesses and their own recoveries will displease everyone with an investment in the current system: the patients, the doctors, and certainly the lawyers who manipulate the health care system like puppeteers. Nevertheless, the new model is needed, and sooner or later everyone will have to wrestle with the changes.

It appears to me that until we adopt the concept that the body is a construction of the spirit and begin to direct medical investigation in a direction different from the current one, medical progress is likely to be stuck at its present level of development. Since development of new concepts is basic to advances in any field of endeavor, it is hard to imagine that many more major improvements in health care can evolve along the lines that medicine has taken thus far. Technology may advance new treatment and diagnostic modalities, but such advancement is not necessarily based upon new concepts. Totally new concepts are always more difficult to evolve and develop than is new technology.

There have been few really new concepts in medicine. Nearly all of the marvelous things we daily read and hear about are technological achievements rather than conceptual developments. All the vaccines and immunizations that have been developed over the years have been extensions of the initial concept of immunization. The Chinese were vaccinating people for smallpox hundreds of years before Jenner got the idea. When Salk and Sabin came up with their polio vaccines, they were great pieces of work, but the idea was not original. The future discovery of a vaccine for AIDS will also be an extension of the original concept. Alexander Fleming was not the first to recognize that penicillin kills certain bacteria, he was just the first to understand the importance of this fact. All the other antibiotics have been spin-offs of his work. Most of what medical science has accomplished has consisted of adaptations of a few important discoveries, like endless movie sequels. This is not to disparage the results of those discoveries and developments, for they appear to have been very helpful, at least on a superficial level. But the greatest breakthrough will come through a totally different concept of humankind and a different model of disease.

When illness occurs, instead of asking the patient what happened to her, we should ask what the illness *means* to her. What she might be hoping to learn or gain from the experience. It is vital that patients' core beliefs concerning their bodies and health be explored. It is here that the cures will be accomplished if they are ever going to be.

Remember that the mind has a close connection via the internal ego with the cells of the body, which have their own consciousness. It must be understood that the internal ego is also in direct communication with the psychological reality of the Universe, called Framework II, while the external ego interacts with society and with the camouflage of reality that is Framework I. Remember, too, that the cells – each with its own consciousness – have the ability to repair and replace themselves without assistance. They can also defend themselves from disease and injury. It has been pointed out in other chapters that beliefs are often implanted in the minds of children concerning their health by parents, peers, and teachers and through other avenues of instruction, such as stories or programs on television. In addition, through the collective memory of the oversoul, recollections of illnesses and injuries can be carried over from one incarnation to another. These beliefs in our own unhealth and disease can quickly become instructions to the bioconsciousness to bring about certain alterations in the basic plan. Conversely, beliefs in vigor, good health, and invincibility augment the cells' natural ability to continue functioning normally. Both kinds of beliefs might be termed core beliefs that set the tone for physical status, just as core beliefs concerning relationships with others, ambitions, attitudes, and the like determine other aspects of our lives.

"Bleed through" memories from other incarnational experiences are not always based on injuries or illnesses from which the person did not recover; memories cut both ways. Other incidents in which injuries healed rapidly and illnesses dissipated swiftly have an impact as well. But these effects are not often investigated. There is, after all, no reason to hypnotize a person who recovered rapidly or to do past life recall to see whether that had been the pattern in other injuries in other lives. If such a study were done, I would be surprised if other life experiences were not found to be just as powerful an influence on the lives of healthy, vigorous individuals.

Secondary beliefs are crucial to the eventual outcome of any health event. Every illness, no matter how mild or insignificant, is potentially fatal, even such a common disease as respiratory infection or intestinal flu. The body defends itself through the wisdom of the cellular consciousness. The individual whose core belief is that he is susceptible to bouts of minor illness does not usually believe he will die from one. His secondary belief concerning his ultimate recovery thereby comes into play, and his cells are instructed, after a time, to exercise their natural ability to recover. These beliefs can be very selective. A person may be certain that he has great resistance to flu yet believe that he is destined to die of cancer, have a heart attack, or develop a kidney disease.

A third factor is often at work in the development of some illnesses. External forces such as toxins, bacteria, viruses, poisons, and other outside elements may, from time to time, overwhelm any individual. But these never act in isolation, for we know that during an epidemic not everyone succumbs to the disease, even though it is reasonable to assume that everyone is more or less equally exposed. As a matter of fact, doctors and nurses often are the most exposed individuals, yet in countless instances they do not become ill. Their immunity may be explained by several elements acting alone or in concert. First, their bodies may be more efficient in defending against the infectious agent. Possibly they have been exposed previously to the disease and still retain some immunity. In addition, their nutrition may be better than that of the general population. There are many reasons why one person will have a better immune system than another. But most important of all, by their intent, health care providers may decide consciously or unconsciously that they cannot afford to become ill. They simply do not have time to be ill and do not allow it to occur.

One of the surgeons under whom I trained was born and raised in central Europe. In the influenza epidemic of 1917, his entire family became ill and several of them died. He told me that, despite the fact that he was not feeling well himself, he continued to work on the family farm and was in the field plowing on the day he became ill. Suddenly, he was seized with a coughing spell and brought up a handful of bright red blood. He said he looked at the blood, wiped his hand on the leg of his trousers, and said to himself, "Well, I guess I have it, too." Then he went on plowing. He laughed as he related the incident, saying that if he coughed up a single drop of blood now, he would be scared to death and immediately have a chest X-ray and a bronchoscopy. Obviously, it had not been his time to die, but his attitude also helped in his recovery. He did not panic, and he did not assume his illness was fatal.

The determination of the cells also plays a critical role in the development of disease. It is crucial to understand that the freedom of choice we assert for the individual human consciousness applies at every level of being. Studies in quantum mechanics have repeatedly shown that quanta, electrons, and atoms have their own sense of purpose and destiny. It is only a small step to understanding that they are each as aware of their individual being as you are of yours. Granted, it is a different kind of awareness, but it is just as intensely focused in its way.

Our society tends to think that only a human being has intelligence, awareness, intent, and understanding of his or her position in the Universe. But this is not so. Every bit of matter and every living thing, plant and animal, has these abilities. Your atoms, molecules, cells, tissues, and organs have certain primary instructions in the form of innate drives and desires that are built into the system. These drives and desires are to remain healthy, to repair themselves, and to cooperate joyfully with the desires of the greater consciousness of which you are a part. *Your cells know what it means to be healthy.* If your core belief urges them to set out on a different course – one of ultimate destruction of the system – the cells are reluctant to comply immediately. It is not that the new commands are considered bad or harmful. It's just that such changes are not made rapidly. There is inertia within the system. Cooperation may be the direction of their intent, but it may take considerable urging on the part of the internal ego to entice them onto a different path.

We commonly see the same thing happening in reverse when it comes to healing. Once the cells alter their behavior to produce a disease process, it often takes multiple instructions over a considerable period of time for them to change their direction. Any doubt or equivocation is taken by the cellular consciousness to question the new instruction and will serve to delay or halt the healing process. Again, inertia is built into the physiological mechanism. Were it not for this lag period, every time we thought of becoming ill, the cells would switch roles. Course changes would be happening so rapidly and frequently as to create total physiologic chaos.

Once the bioconsciousness has altered its purpose to produce or allow an illness, a number of outcomes are possible. The body may recover after a period of time. When it is determined that the body has been sick long enough (whatever that may mean, for the decision is made on an individual basis) the cells will accept a new command not to die and to allow recovery to ensue. Following their internal knowledge and wisdom, the cells know how to accomplish the healing process. This can be done with or without the help of medicine or surgery, although these external forms of assistance may be very helpful in hastening the final result.

The opposite goal may also be reached: death. These plans and decisions are made by the internal ego working within the intertwining events in that measureless labyrinth of spiritual purpose called Framework II. At times, we witness individuals dying of ordinarily nonfatal conditions, and we wonder why. I know of one girl who decided to commit suicide by shooting herself in the head. She was very intent upon dying and did so despite the fact that the bullet only grazed her scalp. There are countless examples of people dying during some minor disease or following some small injury. In these cases, there is usually some insignificant finding that the pathologist will list on the autopsy report and the death certificate. But it is rarely the cause of death, any more than the bullet that grazed the young girl's scalp.

What, then, is the cause of these deaths? Remember, when an individual chooses to die, she will do so. As in all deaths, the spirit simply leaves the body and does not return. These baffling situations simply result from the individual's seizing upon whatever situation or condition is most handy. We view death as tragic and life sacred only because of our intense focus on our biologic lives. This focus tends to blind us to the apparent truth that our lives and our deaths are orchestrated for the purpose of learning various things. As we plan our lives in the reality of Framework II we are aware of this vaster view of life and death. At the level of our deep psychological being, there is no onus to dying.

Between death and recovery lies the chronic state. I have had patients who walked through life arm in arm with their sciatica or their whiplash injury. Their infirmity became so much a part of their personality that it was like having a Siamese twin. Think about this the next time you see someone wearing a cervical collar or a back brace because of an injury sustained months or years before. Think about all the things they may be gaining, or perhaps learning, or missing. Imagine yourself with a cervical sprain and think about what benefits you might accrue by being chronically "injured."

I recall one man in my practice who had a peptic ulcer. He was a sad little guy with a small income and a big family. He would take his ulcer medicine until the pain subsided and then stop the medication. In a few weeks the pain would recur and he would again come to me with his symptoms, acting as though he had no idea what might be causing his indigestion. I would ask whether he was taking his ulcer medicine. Invariably, he would say something like this: "No, I quit taking it several weeks ago. Gee, do you think that's what is causing my heartburn and indigestion? Should I restart the medicine?" Again, I would tell him to resume taking it and not to stop. He would promptly recover, and in a few weeks we would play the game all over again. Clearly, this man was unable to cope with life without the crutch of his ulcer. No doubt he also enjoyed the attention and advantage that having the ulcer afforded him. For one thing, he kept his wife perpetually upset. If he did not wish to do a certain thing, go to work, for instance, his ulcer became a marvelous excuse. If he wanted to engage in certain activities, he was viewed as the martyr who forged ahead in spite of his ulcer. A little illness is truly a wonderful thing to have if you are afraid of life.

Let me present one case that is a perfect representation of this paradigm concerning both the formation of a disease and its cure. One of my best friends, Greg Satre, experienced a horrible childhood full of physical and mental torture and abuse from his stepfather and his mother who orchestrated the abuse and participated as well. His stepfather did not confine his activities to Greg but abused Greg's sisters and brothers as well. He managed to hide his activities by threatening to kill their mother should the children tell her of the abuse. The children were perfectly convinced that he would do just that. During one of his insane episodes, he killed Greg's little sister and was able to pass it off as an accident. Greg knew exactly what had happened, but he was afraid and very isolated, since they lived on a ranch many miles from the nearest neighbor. Furthermore, he felt totally powerless. To atone for his inability to do anything at this horrible moment in his life, Greg made a vow that he would help any person who ever came to him for aid, regardless of the personal effort and sacrifice required or the consequences for him.

That was quite a vow for a young boy to make, but Greg lived up to it. He dedicated his entire life to the vow, extending himself to help everyone he could. The help usually took the form of counseling people who were alcoholics or addicts or who had been physically or sexually abused.

Years passed, and the psychological strain on him became unbearable. He was financially drained and exhausted, literally killing himself both physically and emotionally as he took on other people's troubles. But he did not know how to give up his childhood vow and still maintain his sense of honor. His entire life had been dedicated to the fulfillment of the commitment to help others unconditionally. But after almost fifty years, Greg could no longer go on. Being a man of great integrity, neither could he abandon his life's obligation. Then, several years ago, his internal ego and his bioconsciousness came to his rescue. They gave him a gift that his external ego could not bear to give. They gave him a cancer of his colon. It was a truly marvelous offering! Now he had a genuinely honorable way to escape from his dilemma. If he died of cancer, no one could accuse him of abandoning his vow.

Once the diagnosis was made by the doctor, Greg never returned for treatment. Instead, he sat himself down, meditated, and looked into his subconscious beliefs. There he discovered the link between the vow and the appearance of the cancer. As soon as the connection was discovered, he meditated for weeks, deciding whether he wanted to die or to live. He knew that if he continued to honor his vow in the way that he had, he surely would die, because he could no longer afford to pour that much energy into sustaining it. His final decision was that there was much he needed to do in other areas of his life. He further decided that his journey was between himself and the Universe, so he told absolutely no one of his cancer.

Over the years, Greg had taught many people how to cure themselves of various ills. He reasoned that if his instructions and methods were valid for others, he could surely cure himself. So he put his life on the line. For the better part of two years he meditated. He carried on with his normal business activities, but his nonworking hours were spent probing his subconscious memories, tracing back through his life, tracking all the psychological connections associated with the vow, and setting out new core beliefs by which to live. All the while, he was talking to his bio-consciousness, giving it instructions to return to its normal pattern of health. As a result, the cancer is gone.

This case history is an eloquent example of the development of a cancer for the purpose of giving a person a way out of an unbearable situation. Such cases are wake-up calls to reevaluate our lives. Greg's doctor no doubt attributed the cancer to lack of roughage in his diet and questioned him, I'm sure, about other members of his family who might have had colon cancer. The standard treatment would have been surgery. But, from the deeper, metaphysical approach to understanding the presence of the cancer, it was a gift from Greg's body to his spirit. It was his passport out of an untenable situation, his opportunity to start over. Greg knew this, and he decided that he had already learned too much to leave now. He needed to find a new way to help others on a broader field of play.

Healing himself required a three-pronged approach. Greg knew that the cancer was a great gift. It was the ultimate attention getter, forcing him to reevaluate his life situation. Knowing that illnesses are opportunities to learn and that "fighting" disease is not the proper approach, he *thanked* his body for the cancer. Next, his healing required that he determine how to discharge his childhood vow in a less stressful way. Third, knowing his body was constantly being rebuilt, he had to instruct his cells to return to their normal genetic pattern of growth. To put it another way, he dipped down into the infinite probabilities in Framework II and selected another path for his life that did not include dying of cancer – at least not then.

Many years ago I had a patient who talked constantly about the stupidity of the department head at his university and his desire to run the department himself. He suffered from severe tension headaches that frequently required me to make a house call in the night or to see him in the emergency room of the hospital. The headaches were severe enough to require injections of morphine or Demerol to control the pain. Other drugs were of no use.

This professor was extremely bright, but I also perceived him to be filled with repressed rage at himself and the world. When I tried to talk to him about the headaches, he became very defensive and would not discuss his problem. Nonetheless, I persisted, and after a couple of years, he agreed to let me hypnotize him. The following information was obtained with the use of hypnosis.

The man came from a broken family. His parents were divorced when he was not quite two, and he went to live with his father. He never saw his mother after his parents separated. Under hypnosis he recalled that she had been a demanding, domineering woman who was insistent upon having her own way. Any slight opposition, on even the most insignificant point, would send her into a rage. Her anger led to her getting a headache and, at that point, her husband would feel sorry for her, and she usually got her way. My patient recalled lying in his crib listening to her scream during these temper tantrums, controlling everyone around her. From observing his mother and imprinting on her attitudes, he assumed that controlling others was important above all else. This became a core belief: that to survive in the world and get what you wanted, it was necessary to go into rages and to use headaches as a technique for control.

As he grew up, he was smart enough not to go into rages, but the headaches seemed an acceptable substitute for the entire process. The trouble was that the headaches did not have the same effect on society as the temper tantrums, but he was bound to keep trying. As a result, the headaches became more frequent and more severe. The hypnosis allowed him to see that his headaches were brought about when his efforts to control were thwarted, or when the department head did not agree with whatever he was doing. We talked about the relationship of his headaches to his need for control, but it did little good. He was unwilling to adopt a different way of addressing the world and his life in particular. He might have developed some chronic illness and controlled others through the mechanism of making them feel guilty if they opposed him, but, in the world as viewed from his childhood, headaches had been successful for his mother and he would stick to the method or die trying. In a sense, holding onto the technique of headaches was the same as Greg's holding onto his vow. Psychological, physical, emotional, and spiritual healing are the same. All these are inseparable and must be in harmony if you want a state of total well-being.

Several years passed and the man moved out of town. One day, I received a long letter from him. He had finally come to grips with his core belief, that he had to control everything and everyone to be happy. He wrote that it had taken a year or so, but he had adopted a new attitude toward life: sitting back, observing, and cooperating with people, rather than attempting to control them. He said things seemed to work out very well, even though they sometimes took directions that he was certain would end in failure. Much to his surprise, most of the time his predictions of failure were wrong. He admitted that his desire to have his own department had not been to run the department well, but to be able to control others. The final paragraph of his letter told that once the new attitude was in place, the headaches disappeared. He added that he now ran his own English department at a small college and was enjoying it immeasurably.

Another very instructive case was that of a woman with asthma. She had been conditioned to have problems breathing when cats were present. As a small child, she often faked crying to get her way, and would continue to sob, making noises with each intake of air. On several occasions this happened when a cat was nearby. Her doctor implanted the idea that the "breathing problem" was asthma, due to an allergy to cat dander. This incorrect statement made by her doctor became a core belief and the basis of instructions to her body. Following several episodes of this sort, her bioconsciousness accepted the directions and dutifully produced a real asthma attack every time she was around a cat. All this was discovered with the use of hypnosis, and through its use I managed to reinstruct her body not to react in this way. One way of looking at this is that the patient had a conditioned reflex and that the reflex was extinguished through the use of hypnosis. This is a valid concept, but the effectiveness was dependent upon her adopting another way of thinking about cats and the cells of her respiratory tract exercising another way of behaving. Her lungs went back to their normal way of acting with one instruction under hypnosis, and the asthma was no more.

Another man, a doctor, was not a patient of mine, but he was a close friend. He had been raised by parents who wanted the best for him. That included being a high achiever in school. Their idea of encouragement was to push him to attain the highest grades and, at the same time, to point out constantly where he could have done even better. They saw this as proper constructive criticism, but their son perceived it as something quite different. He saw himself as never quite measuring up to their expectations. In short, he pictured himself as a total failure. No matter how good he was, he was never good enough. As a result of their pushing he went into medicine.

Unfortunately, he married a woman who was much like his mother in that she demanded more than he could possibly give. She was only interested in money and social position. She assumed that, by marrying a doctor, she would have both those things. He was a gentle, introverted person who was anything but a social lion. He preferred to stay home and enjoy his family. Although he made an excellent income, it was not enough to satisfy his wife. My friend was miserably unhappy and insecure and felt himself a hopeless failure. He wanted out, but his love for his children would not allow him to leave. He did not know what to do. His wife was a master at the technique of bait and switch. If he took time off from his practice to participate in family life, his income dropped and she complained, insisting he work longer hours. If he worked long hours, she complained that he should spend more time with the family. Obviously, it was a no-win situation for the doctor. But his cellular consciousness knew exactly what to do and presented him with a heart attack at the age of forty-seven.

The heart attack offered several avenues of relief. First, it could be a stimulus for his wife to show some love and support for him. If she quit her gadding about and reconnected with her husband then it would mean that he was worth something to her after all. Unfortunately, her response to his illness was blame and hateful retribution for the trouble he caused her by interrupting her social life. Once he returned from the hospital to recuperate, she was rarely home. She spent her days eating out with her friends and playing bridge at the country club while he tried to cook his own low-salt meals the best he could.

Before his heart attack he had talked with me on several occasions about leaving town and losing himself, but that was not an option that left him with any self-respect. The heart attack, in contrast, was honorable. Society could not think of him as being a quitter or a failure if he became ill. He was uncertain just what to do, so he allowed himself to survive to think it over.

The attack was a signal for him to reevaluate his life. It was his big opportunity. If he were to continue in the vein of considering himself worthless, then he might as well die and start over rather than waste his time in this way of living. This was his big chance to assert himself and declare his worth and his importance to the Universe. He made a considerable effort. He recovered and returned to his practice, spending many hours at work in an attempt to recover the income lost during his illness.

About a year later, he came home one evening to find that his wife had literally disappeared, leaving him and their children. That was the final blow. He held on several more years, making certain that there was enough money for his children to finish college, and then died of his second heart attack.

In many ways, his parents had helped create the setting for the heart attacks by unwittingly implanting the idea that he was not good enough. His participation, by accepting their suggestions, made it worse. He had the option of rejecting those concepts. No one is obligated to think badly of himself just because others seem to feel that way about him. In this sense, the heart attack was a gift to force him to make a decision. If he were not to change, then further participation in this life was pointless.

Certain life situations can direct a life one way or another, but the final choice is up to you. You are responsible for your own actions, attitudes, and beliefs – and thereby, for your own health. At times, our beliefs are not well thought out and our actions are poorly planned, but blame or fault should not enter the question. It is all a matter of learning. If you give your child a choice between eating her broccoli or her dessert, is she to blame if she makes an unwise choice? How much more secure she will be when she learns and acts upon the truth of her own value of being.

CHAPTER SEVEN

VALUE-FULFILLMENT

IN THE PREVIOUS CHAPTER, we learned that illness is the result of spiritual energy not being given a proper outlet, conflicted and constrained in such a way that the soul is unable to fulfill its greatest constructive potential. Since we are spiritual beings, endowed with an innate desire to enjoy a cooperative interaction with others and the Universe, strife develops deep within us when we are not true to those inherent drives. We find ourselves in turmoil, and this discord is often manifested by mental or physical illness.

The concept of value-fulfillment has no one definition, for it is individually determined first by each species and again by the individual within the species, be it plant, animal, or human. The term implies attainment of a quality of life that goes beyond mere existence and survival. Value-fulfillment entails the ability to add to one's existence a quality of personality, or of character extending beyond the minimum. This is so important to the consciousness' exploration of every living entity that plants and animals will not survive or reproduce in an environment devoid of the elements they feel are necessary to make life worth living. The mere basics of water, food, and shelter may fall far short of their needs.

Value-fulfillment is measured by the depth and intensity of life's experiences – a vastness of being – rather than in the broadness of involvement. It doesn't entail a frantic effort to belong to every organization or be involved in every activity.

Nor is fulfillment reachable through the acquisition of power, influence, wealth, social position, clothes, fine automobiles, or homes in the "right" neighborhood. Everywhere we turn, however, materialism is reinforced. Every advertisement reasserts that acquisitiveness is the proper goal of humankind. But it is possible to possess many things and still be discontented with your life. In fact, material possessions often get in the way of our search for value-fulfillment.

Happiness is elusive and impossible to define or attain. It is not a destination, but a by-product of our seeking value-fulfillment. When I practiced medicine in Champaign, I had a number of university students and their families as patients. Daily, I would listen to them complain that they were unhappy and depressed. The focus of their discontent usually centered on things they wanted and did not have. They would list a washer and dryer, a better car, a larger apartment, a carpet, and so on. For them, happiness was dependent upon satisfying certain conditions: possessing things they wanted. I tried to help them understand that contentment in life could not be conditional, for the moment their conditions were met, another list would be forthcoming. I attempted to lead them to the truth that there is no limit to the number of things one can desire and that the ability to collect them is limited only by one's financial resources. I explained that their lives must have meaning that very day, in the particular circumstances in which they found themselves, or happiness would never be achieved. Most would reply, "Yes, but if I only had. . . ."

When we do not actively seek value-fulfillment, problems arise in our personal lives, our families, our communities, and our nations. When social interactions become skewed, individuals often become mentally or physically ill. At times, the immediate cause of this illness is the futile attempt to emulate others. But each life serves a unique purpose that cannot be assumed by another. No one can possibly fulfill the purpose or function of another human being, nor can we fulfill our souls in imitation of one another.

Living our lives guided by a desire to gain approval from others is just as futile and unrewarding. Looking outside ourselves for validation places us at the mercy of others' expectations. And their approval may or may not come. If the sanction of others is our goal, then we must perform our every action in such a way as to gain outside approval. When we dance to another's tune, we cannot realize value-fulfillment, for we must constantly listen for a change in rhythm and try to keep in step with the other's beat. We become as marionettes on a string and are prevented from creating our own dance.

One of the keys to health and healing is listening to our inner feelings and cooperating with the Universe. We know coming in that we are here to learn and that our first allegiance is to ourselves. At the same time, we know we should be thoughtful and considerate of others. We are aware, for instance, that such attitudes as hate and prejudice are not admirable and should not be tolerated in ourselves. In short, we know what kind of people we should be, and when we are not acting according to those tenets, our spirits are troubled, because we are shut away from inner awareness. As spiritual beings, we are intended to look inward for satisfaction and meaning in life. We have created a society in which wealth and power appear to be personal and even national goals. Common sense tells us that neither of these things is fully attainable. There is no limit to the amount of wealth one can amass, and power is addicting to the degree that no amount is ultimately satisfying.

It is obvious that our bodies are indeed creations of our psyche. Any interference with our quest to attain value-fulfillment will result in some aberration in our physical being. A good example of this is my friend who could no longer fulfill his childhood vow.

Finding himself at a spiritual impasse, his spiritual energy conflicted, his body offered him a solution. Thus, people who are not fulfilling their spiritual purpose, who are not accomplishing what was intended, usually become ill in time. Often the illness is not initially fatal, giving them the opportunity to make adjustments in their lives. At other times, people may be so locked into certain patterns of behavior, or into fulfilling the expectations of others, that they find it impossible to shift probabilities. In these situations, the person may choose to die and start again.

I know another man who was presented with a mild heart attack as a signal to reevaluate his beliefs and prejudices. He is struggling today to restructure his psychological footing and avoid another attack. If he continues in his present attitude toward life, with his heart full of hatred, then further participation on this plane will be of little value. You will recall that people who are contented have little risk of sustaining a cardiovascular catastrophe. Only if we seriously desire to understand what is happening in our lives and to attain some degree of value-fulfillment can our lives be filled with vigor and health.

Ultimately, what we all seek is value-fulfillment: that extra meaning to life that lies beyond mere existence. We aspire to this whether we are aware of it or not. Deep within, every person has certain singular, spiritual desires that he or she wishes to satisfy. We are actually speaking of value-fulfillment when we say that each of us bears his or her own unique gift to the Universe. Life consists of more than being born, growing up, getting an education, getting married and making a home, or working at some job until retirement, and death, overtakes us. It is also more than the collective experiences that occur along the way. Among other things, we are alive for the purpose of adding to the quality of life itself – a quality that is unique in each of us.

We are meant to do this not only as individuals but as members of families, communities, and nations. Whenever we fail to enrich life, we find signals everywhere that point to our deficiency: wars, social upheavals, inconsistent political policies, dysfunctional families, and personal physical and mental illness. Adding to the meaning and value of life is never a static exercise; it is a trial and error process. As we mature, various attitudes and activities must be tried and tested on the scales of reality, and we must cleave to those that prove valuable and abandon those that do not satisfy our intent.

If, as individuals, we hesitate or hold back, fearing that our efforts will not be successful, or in an attempt to save our efforts for a more propitious time, then we will find our lives lacking in luster and spiritual satisfaction. Even more disastrous are moments when we willfully, and at times with evil intent, go against the very nature of our being, abusing others and violating principles of cooperation and peace. When we are not fulfilling our basic intent, very often the warning sign that our lives are not in order will be some illness or injury. These incidents serve as beacons, signaling us to pay attention and reevaluate our beliefs, our values, our goals, and the style in which we conduct our lives. The idea of value-fulfillment includes a quality or depth of action or belief. And quality implies a spiritual intensity – a vastness of being – more than anything else.

We are intended to hold ourselves in high regard, using this standard in our treatment of others. The individual who does not see himself as lovable and as a valued asset to the Universe likely will not have the ability or the courage to extend himself to seek a higher level of awareness, a greater love for his fellow man, or stretch beyond "his place" in society, leaving the Universe a bit better for his having been here.

Value-fulfillment is attainable by every living being. It is sought by every plant, animal, and human. Indeed, even the atoms that compose the Universe seek value-fulfillment at their level of being and awareness. Just to exist is not enough. Creatures who do not strive to attain a vaster consciousness find themselves stunted, constrained, and despondent. Seeking value-fulfillment does not require wealth, social position, or power. Often simple acts of kindness and consideration are sufficient, especially when those acts are not ordinarily required by society. One can always help a friend merely by listening to his problems and helping him sort out the options available to him. Even a smile and a kind word add to the meaning of life, for both giver and receiver.

Part of value-fulfillment is a sense of contentment – a sense that we are spiritually intact and one with the Universe. We know happiness is not an attainable goal except for brief moments in time. But contentment and a peek into one's inner self can be attained through the most elementary activities. Any Buddhist will tell you that a simple, repetitious act of doing the dishes can allow you to focus your attention and gain inner awareness. It is through experiencing inner awareness that we may begin to recognize a sense of our completeness within the Universe, marking the beginning of value-fulfillment.

If you want to experience inner awareness directly, then the autonomous reflex system, the survival reflex of the cellular consciousness, must be reinstructed. Since the system works through the ego energy, the ego must be reinstructed first. This cannot be done by intellect alone and cannot be done by leading with the ego, no matter how powerful and brilliant your intellect, how good and loving your intent, how hopeful your will. And just modifying the ego won't do it either. The ego must be reassured and reinstructed, and this may have to occur initially from a truly childlike stance. Otherwise, the destructive inner connections will, for the most part, remain intact.

Awareness cannot be memorized. The flow of consciousness must be experienced, first through emotion, color, sound, and inner vibrational touch. This process initially can have no agenda except for the experience itself. *After* the experience, after *wordless* reflection, then the intellect may be given permission to relate the experience to the concept. But to get the experience, the ego must be persuaded to surrender to it. The *perceptive* talents of the mind must in every detail replace the autonomous functions of the ego. The intellect is not a perceptive talent but rather an organizational and analytic talent, which is in almost no way the same thing.

In matters of inner awareness, in living it, the intellect must follow, not lead. What opens the doors is to experience, as if for the first time, the song of a bird, the splash of water, the whisper of the wind, the taste of a twig, the texture of a tree, the heat of the sun, the purr of a cat, the resonance of a bell, and to feel the profound innate desire every human being originally has for the opportunity to experience consciousness in these ways.

In order to get some handle on your inner self, a couple of simple exercises can help you feel and become aware of your being and the Universe about you. These are exercises through which you may perceive the world differently.

The first exercise is to center yourself in the energy of the Universe. Everything is energy, and those who are gifted in ways that allow them to see energy patterns tell me they see it happening. The goal, however, is only for you to *feel* it happening. Stand facing north with your eyes closed and your hands at your sides with your palms turned outward. Sweep your arms slowly up to the level of your shoulders. While doing so, imagine and feel yourself pulling the Earth's energy up about you. Imagine that you are now standing in a bowl of golden energy. Pause a moment to imagine, and feel, its presence. Then continue to raise your arms upward slowly until your fingers touch above your head. Now, imagine and feel that you are enclosed in a complete sphere of golden energy. Turn your face upward with your eyes still closed. After a moment or two, spread your arms a bit, opening the top of the sphere, letting the energy from the Universe in. Imagine and feel and "see" it as a shaft of brilliant blue or white light. Then say the words "I am." After another moment or two, turn your palms outward again and sweep your arms down to your thighs as though you were swimming. Imagine the surge of energy as you sweep downward and feel the sensation of lightness, almost as though you were being lifted from the floor. Finally, anchor yourself by bringing your arms up to shoulder level again. At this point, feel yourself eternally authenticated in space and time. Feel that you truly belong here and are totally acceptable as a human being. Open your eyes and appreciate the experience. Do not attempt to analyze your feelings or explain them in any way.

The second exercise is a Zen Buddhist one that perhaps is more intellectual. Sit quietly in a chair and think of your position as being in the center of a circle – perhaps the hub of an invisible wagon wheel. Extending from the center of the circle into space about you are any number of spokes, as numerous as required for your exercise. Mentally push everything with which you are involved out along the spokes to the periphery of the circle, out to the rim of the wheel. Place there, in the outer circle, your spouse, children, parents, relatives, in-laws, friends, house, possessions, religion, social position, job, hobbies, desires, accomplishments, ambitions, convictions, others' beliefs about you, your health, beliefs about your health, and everything you have learned at this level. Place everything – all ego attachments – out in the circle. Experience the truth that those things, people, ideas, beliefs, concepts, and attachments are not *you*.

Once this experience is attained, feel yourself – the real you – unattached and free. Feel the wonder of your own validity. The test of your success in gaining this new stance would be your equanimity if someone came to you saying that your spouse and children were all killed when your car ran into your house, and that the house has burned to the ground. Your relatives, in-laws, and friends have abandoned you. Your savings are lost and you were just fired. The doctor called saying you have but a month to live. The church excommunicated you, and you have just discovered that everything you have learned and believed has been proven false. At this point, if you have truly reached the *ultimate* objective of the exercise, you could say, "So far, nothing has happened to me. My essential being is intact!"

At this point, you are free to become involved with life, but the involvement will no longer be at an ego level. Your ego will no longer be on the line. If something goes awry, you will be able to acknowledge it without feeling guilty or attempting to place blame. Thus free, you are able to set about fixing it. As far as your health is concerned, you will know that your body is only a possession. After all, only your body is ill. Centered, you are empowered to change your beliefs, habits, attitudes, or whatever is required to release the flow of your healing energy.

When he was living in Japan, the German physician and author Karlfried Graf von Durkheim was asked an interesting question by a Zen Buddhist master. The master had been looking at a painting by a Bavarian artist that Graf von Durkheim had hanging in his apartment. The old man asked, "Wasn't the artist through?" Graf von Durkheim did not know what he meant by the term "through." The master replied, "Wasn't he beyond all fear of death?" "Wasn't he consumed by love for all of the Universe?" and "Wasn't he able to see the sense beyond the nonsense of life?" In many ways, these questions strike at the heart of the meaning of value-fulfillment. It is by understanding death that we lose our fear of it. Certainly, love is the most valued emotion, the one that reaches beyond all others. But understanding that we cannot appreciate one value without its opposite being present to act as a benchmark is critical. Accepting this concept leads us to be less judgmental toward others and ourselves. It puts our reactions beyond the level of placing blame and guilt and exacting punishment. These qualities of personality, love and nonjudgmental understanding, free us to pursue value-fulfillment and, thereby, health and fullness of being.

I can attest that as I incorporated metaphysical concepts into my belief system, a great many events the purpose of which I had not understood before became clear to me in light of my newfound knowledge.

Recently, I was asked how it feels to be healthy. I had never been asked this question before, nor had I ever had one of my patients offer any statements along that line, even when they had just recovered from some illness. Except for a minor cold or two and a sore wrist and shoulder years ago, I have not been ill for almost sixty years. Physically, I feel as good as I have at any time in my life. I am as agile as when I was forty. I become sleepy at bedtime, but rarely am I tired. I awaken in the morning fresh and invigorated, having slept soundly. My appetite is good, too good. I go about my daily activities with cheerful enthusiasm. I have learned to see the sense beyond the nonsense of life.

Emotionally, I am satisfied with my life. I have no regrets. That is not to say that I have not done a few stupid things or made some poor decisions. But I know these things happen to all human beings, and I am no exception. I have never allowed guilt to be part of the process, nor have I accepted blame for my actions. I have simply taken responsibility and then made an effort not to repeat the mistake.

Each day I enjoy the confidence that comes from knowing that I am one with the Universe. I know well that I will have ample time to accomplish anything the Universe has in mind for me to do. I have never in my life had the slightest fear of death. In fact, I have always felt death to be the ultimate adventure of life. This is not morbid. It is simply an affirmation that death does not really occur, except to the body. And when my time is up, I have full confidence that entities wiser than I will have helped me engineer the plan in detail.

But more important is the knowledge that I am acceptable in every way to the Universe, and that my spiritual being and my physical being are unified and at peace. Through the years, I have made a concerted effort to add to the quality of my life through my interaction with others and my continual search for knowledge and wisdom that lie beyond the normal parameters of the traditional educational goals of a physician.

And I owe my good health to the long years I've known these things and have fortified myself with these truths.

PART

TWO

THE TREATMENT OF ILLNESS AND THE RETURN OF HEALTH

CHAPTER EIGHT

COMPARISON OF HOLISTIC AND STANDARD MEDICINE

I AM SURE THAT some of you are struggling to understand how a new belief system will fit in with the old, obsolete models of caring for ourselves when we are hurt or ill. The first step is to understand that adversity, not peace of mind, prompts us to discover new vistas of knowledge. Karlfried Graf von Durkheim spoke with me of the process of enlightenment while we were attending a conference in northern Italy in 1961. Graf von Durkheim described it as an experience in which the individual attempts to gain wisdom while remaining uncertain that anything is being accomplished or learned. Eventually some signal event will occur in her life. It may be an illness, perhaps something that frightens her, a sudden confrontation of some sort, or a natural catastrophe. Whatever the incident, the person will realize abruptly that she has arrived at a higher plane of enlightenment than she previously occupied.

In the awareness of her newfound station, she can look back, for a moment, at her former level of being and appreciate the progress she has made. Then, as she becomes involved with her daily activities, she will lose sight of her newly attained position until another incident occurs, perhaps years later. Thus it is that we learn, *or* if you prefer, gain enlightenment, in quantum jumps. We gain knowledge as bits and pieces are collected by our minds in what can only be termed packets.

These are stirred around in our thoughts until suddenly we comprehend them as an integrated whole. It is the comprehension of the integrated whole that we call wisdom. Rarely can we assimilate large blocks of new information at once. But the intellect will accept one packet of understanding at a time so that, through our intellectual struggles, we can prepare ourselves to make a quantum jump into a vaster orbit of wisdom.

The other day, I was asked by a friend to help her daughter with a science project. The girl had tackled quite a problem. She sought to correlate stress with the development of illness in older people. They asked me to look over the list of illnesses that were, according to standard, accepted medical thinking, due to stress and see whether I could think of diseases to add. I read over the list and found myself confused. None of the conditions or diseases listed seemed to fit the model of being caused solely by stress. Certainly, stress contributes to every medical condition, but is it the cause?

Ulcerative colitis, I knew, was due to unexpressed outrage and anger and triggered by a maladaptive food reaction. Multiple sclerosis and eczema were due to reactions to various foods. High blood pressure was related directly to sodium in the diet. All the conditions on the list resulted *from* a desire of the spirit to become ill, or at the very least the willingness to cooperate in the event, *for* whatever reason. I shook my head, read over the list, and tried again. For a moment I could not fathom why I was having such difficulty. Then I realized that I was having trouble getting back into the old mechanistic mode of thinking that is normal *for* the majority of doctors. I had so completely altered my belief system concerning the paradigm of illness and disease that I was unable to shift readily back into the thought patterns I had learned in medical school.

Later, as I was reflecting on the incident, I became amused at my mental block. I realized that asking physicians and patients who may not have had any thoughts along these lines quickly to alter their belief system and accept the new model would cause them as much confusion as I expcrienced when I attempted to think in the old way. I remember a few years ago when Greg Satre and I were discussing a metaphysical problem as it related to medicine. I grasped the concept in the abstract, but when I attempted to apply it to my medical practice my mind balked. I recall shaking my head in puzzlement and saying, "Wait a minute. This is counter to everything I learned in medicine. Give me some time to integrate this concept."

During the forty-four years I practiced medicine, I made a sincere attempt to lead my patients toward an eclectic approach to their illnesses as I learned each new bit of information and gained skill in that direction. It was not easy for them, and a surprising number were totally uninterested in pursuing new approaches to their health, no matter how promising the results might be. They didn't want to be involved beyond taking a few pills, and much less did they feel they might be responsible for the development of their illnesses, or for their recovery. They would look at me and say something to the effect that it was *my* responsibility to get them well. I was, after all, the doctor. Just give them a prescription and dispense with all the talk. I learned that the majority of patients were completely dissatisfied with me if they did not leave my office with a prescription in hand. Without some tangible evidence of their visit, the perception was that I had not done anything for them.

We all must make the effort to change – if not now, then soon. And change, when it comes seeping through the cracks of our faulty notions of health and disease, will probably require several generations to be fully accepted. To that end, it may be helpful to consider several examples of medical problems and compare the standard approach with the newer eclectic paradigm. The following are not hypothetical cases. They represent actual medical cases of patients I had or with whom I am familiar.

Bill was almost fifty years old. For the last several years, he had had chest pains from time to time. They were not bad pains, more like a dull ache in the middle of his chest. His wife had nagged him to get a physical, so he finally went to his doctor and had "the works. "

On questioning, Bill revealed that his father had died at the age of forty-seven from a heart attack. One of his uncles had a heart attack when he was thirty-eight and died of his second coronary at the age of fifty-three. The history further brought out that Bill smoked two packs of cigarettes a day. The laboratory tests showed his cholesterol to be 276, the fasting blood sugar was 138, and his blood pressure was elevated at 164/92. An EKG was performed. It was normal, except for a slight depression of the ST segments in his lateral chest leads, which indicated some mild left ventricular strain. He was five feet, eight inches tall and weighed 197 pounds.

According to the Framingham study conducted at Harvard medical school, he was at extremely high risk for some cardiovascular catastrophe. All these factors were present: male, a smoker, systolic hypertension, glucose intolerance, high cholesterol, and evidence of electrocardiographic changes. In addition, his doctor noted his family history of coronary artery disease. Bill was scheduled for an EKG treadmill test the next day. It demonstrated a three-millimeter drop in his ST segments upon moderate exercise associated with some substernal chest pain.

Bill was admitted to the hospital that night and the next morning was subjected to coronary arteriography. The X-rays revealed a 75 percent block midway down his anterior descending coronary artery. The surgeon was called in and, after a brief discussion, Bill was scheduled for a balloon angioplasty. Two days later in the operating room, a catheter with a tiny balloon was inserted into his coronary artery and the fatty deposit was compressed, thereby relieving the obstruction. Bill was told that everything had been taken care of.

Following his hospitalization, his doctor handed him a low cholesterol diet sheet. He told Bill to lose weight, to cut down on his salt intake, and to stop smoking. The doctor also prescribed a diuretic to lower his blood pressure. At every office visit his doctor lectured him on the importance of losing weight and stopping smoking, saying that if Bill did not follow directions, he would have a heart attack and die before he retired. Seventeen months after his angioplasty, while on his way to work one Monday morning, Bill ran into the back of the car ahead of him that had stopped at a traffic light. He was found slumped over the steering wheel, dead. An autopsy showed that the fatty plaque had recurred and was blocking 90 percent of the blood flow. However, there were no changes in the heart muscle to indicate that he had actually sustained a heart attack.

His doctor was surprised to learn of Bill's death. He had thought that everything was going along well. Bill had cut his smoking down to one pack and had lost eight pounds. His blood pressure was down to 152/90 and his cholesterol was 245. Bill had claimed that he felt fine when the doctor had seen him last. The doctor justified his medical management of Bill, saying that at least he had done all the proper things and given him another seventeen months with his timely medical intervention.

Down the street from his office was a holistic clinic. Bill's doctor did not think much of its staff, for they were a strange bunch with strange ideas. He had even heard that some patients who went there did not necessarily see either of the two doctors but were treated by some of the other people on the staff. He had learned that they had a full-time nutritionist and a chiropractor working there, and it was rumored that sometimes a hypnotist and an acupuncturist came in as well. At the county medical society meeting, they had discussed the fact that one of the doctors had received training in homeopathy. Although there was little they could do about it, none of the doctors at the meeting was pleased at having the clinic in their midst. No, Bill's doctor had nothing to do with them nor they with him, and he was glad.

The clinic was treating a man whose situation was almost identical to Bill's. The two patients were only a year apart in age and had the same medical problems, but Ted's treatment was quite different from what Bill had experienced. The clinic's approach to his problem was based upon a different system of beliefs and priorities.

Ted presented himself to the clinic's doctor with a complaint of chest pain. During the taking of the history, the doctor asked about his relatives. At the doctor's urging, Ted talked a great deal about how he felt when his father died of a heart attack at a young age. The doctor inquired in depth concerning Ted's beliefs about heart attacks and whether he had assumed that he would die from one too. Ted admitted that he had read all he could about heart disease occurring in families, but he had not discussed it with his wife. The doctor also asked about his lifestyle. What did he like to eat? How much did he smoke? What did he do for fun? Did he have a dog or cat? Did he like his job? How many hours a week did he work? What kind of relationship did he have with his boss? Was he exhausted at the end of the day? Did he get along well with his wife and kids? Was he happy, or was life drudgery? Then the physician ran a battery of laboratory tests and did an EKG, which indicated a condition similar to Bill's. Ted's cholesterol was 270, his blood sugar 140, and his blood pressure 168/94.

After the test results were received, Ted was directed to the nutritionist. Noting that his blood sugar indicated a mild diabetes, she tested Ted for a food intolerance and found that he reacted to corn. She incorporated that fact into the special diet she prescribed, eliminating all corn and corn products. Ted's wife was included in the process. Both she and Ted were instructed in the preparation of tasty, very low sodium, low saturated fat meals that did not contain corn products. He was also placed on a multiple vitamin-mineral tablet with additional potassium and magnesium supplements. Two weeks later, another blood sugar revealed the fasting level to be down to 102 and blood pressure at 134/74. Ted volunteered that the chest pain was gone.

In the meantime, one of the clinic members began working with Ted toward changing his core belief structure concerning death and heart attacks. With his guidance, Ted began to realize that he had assumed he would die of a heart attack as his father had. All his life, he had heard how much alike they were. In fact, his father had been his role model, and Ted attempted to emulate his father in every way. Eventually, Ted came to grips with the idea that dying as his father had was a hidden expectation he had adopted. The therapist helped him understand that, simply because he had accepted his father as a person to imitate, he did not have to go so far as to die at the same age. Gradually, Ted came to comprehend that it was possible to choose another probability for his life that did not lead to death at the age of fifty.

The physician who had done his original history and physical hypnotized Ted several times and managed to help him quit smoking. A month after his first examination, Ted was still pain free. A repeat EKG was normal. His blood pressure was 126/68, and life seemed a lot better. Ted began to read some metaphysical literatuie suggested to him by the therapist. It was a bit confusing at the start, but as he read and thought about it, he had to admit that it made sense. He learned, through his reading and with the help of the therapist at the clinic, that he created his life and his body through his belief system. He began to look at his job in a different light. One day, Ted suddenly realized that nearly all of the things he hated most about his job were of his own making. He saw the humor of the situation and set about creating a different environment. He quit taking things so seriously and found himself laughing just from the sheer enjoyment of it all.

Ted died at the age of sixty-two. He had given himself twelve years of joyful living. He had learned the lesson brought into focus by his chest pain. His threatened heart attack had truly been a wonderful gift, bringing as it did an understanding to his life while teaching him to accept responsibility for his own fate. That was what it had all been about. The impending heart attack had been a gift, forcing Ted into a position where he had either to take charge of his own life or to continue to abrogate his responsibility. In choosing the best path of action, Ted had given himself another twelve years to enjoy the fruits of his efforts.

At a deep spiritual level, Ted knew all of this. He died knowing that he had fulfilled his learning mission. Since Ted had nothing to learn from a slow and painful death, he subconsciously chose to leave while doing something that he loved. He and his wife were hiking through the mountains. It was a beautiful fall day, the last day of their vacation, and the foliage was at its peak of color. Ted was standing near the edge of a cliff enjoying the view. He turned away from the scene and remarked to his wife that it was one of the best days of his life. As he turned back to look again, his heel slipped on a rock, and he fell over the precipice. Before his body hit the rocks far below, the spirit detached itself and glided away to another dimension.

The standard approach to an impending heart attack is purely mechanistic, based upon the belief that heart attacks are caused solely by a blockage of the blood flow to the heart muscle. Physicians are aware that other factors enter in, such as high blood pressure, diabetes, high cholesterol, and smoking. But they see these factors as contributing to the development of the cholesterol plaques that block the arteries. They do not see a heart attack as a spiritual/ social/nutritional cellular disease in which the blocked artery plays only a minor role. To his doctors, Bill's condition was a mechanical problem to be approached by mechanical methods. Following his balloon angioplasty, Bill was placed on a diuretic to treat his high blood pressure despite the fact that diuretics cause the heart cells to lose potassium, thereby increasing the chance for an abnormal rhythm in the heart and an often fatal electrical event. The doctor's aim was to lower Bill's pressure by a simple means. The strategy was effective, but the potassium loss probably contributed to Bill's cardiac arrest.

Bill's early adult onset diabetes was not addressed because his doctor felt that Bill's blood sugar was not sufficiently high to warrant medication. Thinking that Bill's weight was the cause of his elevated fasting blood sugar, the doctor prescribed a reducing diet. Then, to make matters worse, he did what most doctors do. He threatened Bill at every office visit, saying that if he did not follow instructions, he would have a heart attack and die. Bill was already under stress from his job, and listening to his doctor preach doom and defeat was the wrong thing for him. Certainly, trying to gain the patient's cooperation is essential, but rather than attempting to educate Bill, the doctor simply abused him.

The physician who treated Ted knew all about risk factors. He did not believe, however, that they constituted the sum total of the issues to be addressed in the treatment of an impending heart attack. As I indicated previously, if a person is happy and enjoys his work, he is far less likely to have a heart attack, regardless of his blood pressure, cholesterol, or any of the other risk factors. Nutrition played a strong role in Ted's treatment, as did bringing him to understand that he had programmed himself to have a heart attack. Learning about the metaphysical aspects of life gave Ted a new footing from which to approach his life. The very low salt diet was sufficient to bring his blood pressure down to normal – that and his learning to handle stress. All in all, the comprehensive approach to Ted's condition proved to be a better way. It was, in fact, the best approach and would have been the best even if it had not been so successful.

This next case is highly instructive in demonstrating how illness can be programmed by our beliefs and attitudes. It also illustrates the value of taking an eclectic approach to illnesses, which often solves many problems that narrower approaches fail to address.

Susan was forty-eight and still troubled with asthma. She had had her first asthmatic attack when she was eighteen months old. It came in the form of a bronchiolitis secondary to a viral infection. After that, every time she got a bad cold, she would wheeze and cough for several weeks. She also developed middle ear effusions that defied treatment. The pediatrician finally referred her to an ear, nose, and throat specialist who placed tubes in her eardrums to allow the mucus to drain away, but it never did. Susan underwent a number of scratch tests for allergies at the age of eight. The tests demonstrated a moderate reaction to molds and dust. As a result of the tests, she was given allergy shots for almost six years, with little apparent improvement. The doctor kept reminding her mother how much worse Susan would be if it were not for the shots.

After Susan became an adult, she no longer had the ear problems, but she was troubled by a postnasal drip that was a constant source of irritation. Various opinions by many doctors were quite contradictory. Some favored more allergy tests and desensitizing injections. Others recommended antihistamines and bronchial dilators. Susan finally settled upon taking an aminophylline medication that relieved the tightness in her chest to some extent.

To the mechanistically oriented physicians she consulted during her life, Susan's case was a rather cut-and-dried affair, despite the ineffectiveness of their treatments. Other than the things they had tried repeatedly, the doctors knew of nothing else to do. They considered prescribing steroids but, since Susan's trouble was not critical, they opted not to go that route.

Susan finally consulted another physician. He listened to her problems and did a thorough examination, which gave him little information except for the sound of a few wheezes in her lungs on deep breathing. Because of the meager evidence in her history to account for her lifelong difficulty, coupled with her poor response to therapy, the doctor decided to hypnotize her. In his experience, when patients failed to respond to good therapy, there was usually some underlying psychic reason for their lack of response. Under deep hypnosis, she returned to her first episode of bronchiolitis. As she began to recall the event, she cried that she was going to die, "just like last time." The doctor then guided her back to the memory of a past life. Susan responded that, in the incarnation immediately preceding this one, she had died of asthma at the age of seven. She said she had suffered one infection after another, complicating her asthma. She lost weight and became weaker with each episode, she said, and ultimately she died. While Susan was still under hypnosis, the doctor brought her forward to the childhood of her present life. Gradually, he helped her realize that this was a different body and that things did not have to repeat themselves. He worked to reassure her bio-consciousness that it did not need to respond to the memories of her other illnesses. As a result of three hypnosis sessions, Susan's wheezing disappeared.

But the doctor was still faced with Susan's problem of the childhood ear effusions and the postnasal drip. Using a chiropractic maneuver, he tested her for a reaction to various common foods. The doctor had Susan hold different foods in one hand while he tested the strength of her other arm. It was quickly evident that when she held dried milk in the palm of her hand, the biceps muscle in her other arm was noticeably weaker. This did not occur when she held any other food. Subsequently, her doctor advised her to refrain from eating or drinking any milk or milk products for a period of ten days. When she returned, she reported that her postnasal drip had vanished and some residual feeling of tightness in her chest had also disappeared.

At the doctor's direction, Susan drank a glass of milk the next morning at breakfast. She ate nothing else. Within twenty minutes, her nose was running profusely and she was wheezing and coughing up a large amount of mucus. By evening of that day, she was again symptom free.

Susan's lifelong medical problems stemmed from an intolerance for cow's milk compounded by the subconscious fear that she would die of asthma. From an early age Susan had instructed her respiratory tract to behave as it had in her other life. Her memory had been triggered by her first episode of bronchiolitis when she was a baby. The cells of her respiratory tract cooperated with the directions of the vaster authority, her internal ego. As a consequence of the comprehensive intervention, Susan now is completely free of her draining mucus and her exertional asthma.

When Jim was playing football in high school, he dislocated his left shoulder. The team physician reduced the dislocation and, after a month, Jim resumed sports without any further difficulty. His shoulder gave him no trouble until he was fifty-three. One afternoon, he was working on his back porch, tripped, and fell down three steps. Jim managed to avoid striking his head on the sidewalk by taking most of the force of the tumble on his left shoulder. In the process, he also bumped his knee and cut the palm of his hand slightly. The next day, his shoulder was a little tender and his knee was very swollen and stiff. He thought little of it, took some ibuprofen, and went on about his business. The knee promptly recovered. But over the next three weeks, his shoulder became progressively painful. He began to lose motion, and the discomfort kept him awake at night. He consulted his doctor.

On examination, an X ray failed to reveal any fracture. Jim's doctor prescribed a number of anti-inflammatory drugs over several weeks, but they did no good. The doctor eventually sent Jim to an orthopedic surgeon, who prescribed yet another anti-inflammatory drug, which also provided Jim no relief. Finally, he admitted him to the hospital and performed arthroscopy. Inserting a tiny telescope into the joint, he found that the capsular tear from the old dislocation had not healed. Finding nothing else to explain the incapacitating pain and loss of motion, he scheduled Jim for a surgical repair of the old joint capsule injury. The surgery was a success, but the symptoms did not abate. By this time it had been almost a year and a half since Jim fell off the porch.

Jim felt he had nothing to lose by seeking another opinion. He approached another doctor who was thought to be quite unorthodox but whose patients swore by him. The new doctor listened to what had transpired. Jim had received all the latest treatment medical technology had to offer and was becoming worse rather than better. On the basis of his experience, the doctor suspected that another life event might be playing a part. He asked Jim to come in to be hypnotized, explaining that, if nothing else, he might be able to control his pain using meditative and self-hypnotic techniques.

Fortunately, he proved to be a good hypnotic subject. The doctor gave him suggestions concerning the pain and demonstrated to Jim how to block pain by picturing himself in a beautiful garden where all is serene and peaceful. With this accomplished, the doctor regressed Jim to the day he fell off the porch. Speaking with him under hypnosis, he asked if he had ever injured either of his shoulders before, an open-ended question with no time constraints. After a bit of urging, in which the doctor suggested that the mind never forgets anything, Jim related an incident in which he had been in the cavalry. He said that he had fallen off a horse and sustained a severe fracture of his shoulder that did not heal. He remained crippled until he died.

There was the connection. The minor injury that Jim sustained when he fell off the porch occurred at about the same age at which he said he had been thrown from a horse. This present injury reminded him of the other injury. His internal ego simply instructed the bio-consciousness of his shoulder tendons, ligaments, and muscles to behave in the same manner as before. The cells cheerfully cooperated with his mental command. Then the doctor instructed Jim's shoulder that it was a different one than before. He further indicated that his present shoulder had long since recovered from the injury he sustained when he fell off the porch and from the surgery. When the hypnosis session ended, the pain was gone. Jim's shoulder was a bit stiff from disuse, but in another few weeks it loosened up to allow a full range of motion.

This is not an unusual situation by any stretch of the imagination. When doctors do all the right things, but they are not adequate to the task, most doctors look for a different pill or therapy. Rarely does it occur to them that their basic assumptions concerning the cause of the condition may be in error. They are not taught to consider that a patient's internal beliefs and thoughts can produce an actual illness or sustain an injury. So doctors, and those who are conditioned to believe their every remark, continue to search for an external cause for every malady. What we should consider is that when a proven medicine is not effective, perhaps medicine is not the answer. It is only by stepping beyond convention that the physician may discover other perfectly legitimate approaches to his patients' problems. By trying an alternate approach, neither the doctor nor the patient burns his bridges. Jim's shoulder could always have been operated upon, but it cannot be "unoperated." By focusing on the old, unhealed injury that was asymptomatic and that was not actually the cause of his pain, the surgeon had performed an unnecessary operation.

When Chuck was fifty-six, his physical examination found nothing to be amiss. He appeared to be in excellent shape. Upon completion of the exam, his doctor ordered him to have a battery of tests, including the new test that had been developed to diagnose early prostate cancer. The doctor had not felt any abnormality in Chuck's prostate, but this test was the newest thing, and he had been urging all his male patients over forty-five to have it performed. Chuck agreed, because he had known an associate who had prostatic cancer, and it had not been a pretty thing. If he had a prostate cancer, he certainly wanted to catch it early so he could be cured.

All the tests came back normal except for the prostate one. His doctor explained that the level of prostate-specific antigen (PSA) was slightly elevated. Not enough to be certain he had cancer, but enough to warrant repeating the test in three months. Chuck was frightened. He did not tell his wife, but he secretly brooded and worried about the cancer he was certain he had. He lay awake at night trying to imagine what it would be like. He was only fifty-six! Would he be able to make love to his wife? After the three months were up, Chuck did not return. He was afraid what the test would reveal. He was certain that he had cancer and did not want to hear the news. His wife finally made him go to the doctor. The test was still slightly elevated but no more conclusive than before. This time, he was told to return in six months.

Chuck was concerned about the long wait. Maybe it was a good sign but, nonetheless, he worried constantly. It did not consume his every thought, but it was never far from his mind. When he went to the bathroom, he watched the flow of urine very carefully, looking for any evidence of decreased power in the stream. He became conscious of many feelings in that part of his body. His common sense told him that he was probably imagining things, that these were feelings he had always had but never before noticed. Still, he worried. He made a new will. As the months passed, Chuck's level of concern subsided to some extent. He still thought a lot about the test, though, and finally decided that if he got a cancer he would just have to face it as he had done other things in his life.

After his next prostate test, the results were the same: slightly elevated. Again the doctor cautioned that the results were not conclusive and that Chuck should not worry. But he did. He didn't sleep that night. He lay awake totally convinced that he had cancer and that the doctor was keeping it from him. He told his wife that the test was normal and buried his fear inside.

At the end of six months, Chuck returned as requested. On rectal examination, the doctor felt something new. There was a stony-hard nodule in the left lobe of his prostate. The doctor was surprised at its size. The prostate test showed a high PSA level consistent with cancer. Chuck received the latest drugs and underwent a radical prostatectomy. Six months later his hip broke as he was walking to the dining room table. The bone scan demonstrated that there were metastases throughout many parts of his skeleton. He died seven months later.

From the metaphysical point of view, Chuck died when his time was up. But we need not view the time of individuals' deaths as being chiseled in stone. Having resigned himself to death, Chuck may have altered his probabilities and accepted death when it might not have been necessary to do so. There is little doubt that the test had given him something to focus his fears upon and a blueprint for illness. Certainly, there is nothing wrong with having tests performed. Chuck's problem came when the tests were inconclusive. The doctor's informing him of the ambiguous results led to Chuck's uncertainty and then to a very specific fear. Chronic anxiety increases the level of cortisol in the body and blunts the defenses to infections and tumors. In this sense, there are times when ignorance is truly bliss. By assuming the attitude that he did, Chuck gave a strong message to his prostate gland that he was expecting a cancer. The unpleasant memories of his associate's difficulty added to his fear. His fear and anxiety literally begged his prostate to comply with his hidden assumption that a malignancy had begun. The bio-consciousness of his prostatic cells had every reason to comply with the subliminal instructions from his internal ego to develop a cancer. As I have said, all the cells in the body exercise their intent in the form of cheerful cooperation with the mind's vaster consciousness, and so Chuck's prostatic cells followed his unspoken orders.

Prostate cancers are known to lie dormant for many years, found only on autopsy after a man dies of some other cause. This might have been the case with Chuck had he not received the test or been told of the uncertain results. As it was, his instructions to his cellular consciousness may well have activated an otherwise quiescent tumor.

An eclectically oriented doctor probably would have run the test but, upon getting a borderline, equivocal result, would consider saying nothing. If it was not time to treat the patient, why worry him? The prostate cancer test could have been followed up in the future without causing anxiety and fear with the explanation that it produced many false and misleading answers or that it was necessary to repeat the test in order to establish each patient's normal value.

153

Had he experienced an ongoing relationship with his patient, the eclectic physician more than likely would have spoken of altering probabilities, and using one's intent to instruct the bio-consciousness in ways of health long before a critical situation presented itself. When the doctor found the tumor or the test results rose, that would be the perfect time to begin helping Chuck examine his core beliefs, and to start reinstructing his cellular consciousness to bring about a change in the cellular configuration of his prostatic cells. Hypnosis, acupuncture, and nutrition could have been used to augment the process. It is obvious that the radical prostatectomy did nothing other than to support the physician's conviction that for cancer he must do something really dramatic. Attention to good nutrition and metaphysical counseling, in conjunction with the latest medicines, would likely have done as much if not more than the surgery. And if the patient opted for surgery, the alternate methods would augment any benefit gained by the operation.

Another man, by the name of Henry, was referred to an eclectically oriented clinic because of a benignly enlarged prostate gland that was blocking his flow of urine. His prostate gland was huge, filling his lower pelvis. Normally, at his age, seventy-four, he would have been a prime candidate for a prostatic resection to relieve the blockage. Henry's problem was that he had just had a sizable heart attack, and there was no way a surgeon was going to subject him to surgery unless it was in response to a life-threatening condition. For this reason, his doctor had sent him to the clinic to see what they might do.

Under the direction of a psychologist, Henry was hypnotized and some suggestions were made to the effect that his prostate was going to shrink to normal size. Then he was taught meditative techniques in which he visualized his prostate becoming smaller. He was told to think of this happening in some manner of his own choosing. Henry decided to imagine his prostate being whittled away by tiny elves working day and night. He practiced this exercise for ten minutes twice a day. Within two days Henry was experiencing some relief, and by ten days his urinary stream had enlarged considerably. On examination his prostate was found to be somewhat smaller. Henry was discharged and told to return in four weeks. In the meantime, he was to continue his visualizations twice daily. Upon his return, Henry's prostate was nearly normal in size.

Henry had intently focused his mind on the problem at hand. Under his own constant barrage of instruction, Henry's prostate gland restructured itself according to his directions. Henry lived another eleven years and never again had trouble with his prostate.

Jane's menstrual periods had always been normal until two days after her forty-second birthday. She began to spot and bleed. She consulted a gynecologist, who did an endometrial biopsy; the results were normal. The doctor told Jane that the bleeding was most likely the result of some tiny fibroid tumors that he had felt during the pelvic exam. He said that a hormone imbalance caused by her impending menopause could also account for the bleeding. For three more months she took various hormones but continued to bleed. Then the doctor talked to her about the need for a hysterectomy. Jane did not want to have her uterus removed but felt that slowly bleeding to death was not a good idea either. At this point she consulted another doctor.

The other doctor had an excellent reputation for solving medical problems that seemed to baffle his colleagues. He listened to Jane's recounting of the events and did a pelvic examination. True, she did have some tiny fibroid tumors, but he believed there were other things to try besides hormones and surgery. He suggested they try hypnosis. He promised her nothing but said only that it might shed some light on the subject. It took a while, but Jane finally achieved a deep trance. He asked her if she had ever had a problem with vaginal bleeding at any other time. Immediately, Jane began to cry. The doctor suggested that she could recall the event without being upset. She stopped crying and related this story.

In her previous life, Jane had been married to a man who dearly loved children. But she had never been able to conceive. Then, at the age of forty-two, she became pregnant. Her husband was elated but she was not. After several days of agonizing she secretly went to an abortionist. Although the fetus was aborted, she had continued to bleed. Her husband had no idea what had happened. The woman was filled with guilt and remorse for her act. She bled for several weeks. By the time her husband intervened and took her to a doctor himself, she had developed an infection. The blood loss coupled with the infection caused her death, and she had died with her soul filled with guilt and grief.

The doctor then led her back hypnotically to her present life, to the weeks before she began to spot. They discussed the event while Jane was hypnotized, and the doctor allowed her to see that punishing herself was unnecessary. He obtained an unequivocal promise from her to stop the bleeding. Then he allowed her to come out of hypnosis.

Jane had no more vaginal bleeding. Her menstrual periods returned to normal, and the depression that she had been experiencing during those months disappeared.

Jane's gynecologist did all the correct things in treating her. He properly ruled out an endometrial carcinoma by doing the biopsy. He attempted hormone therapy before suggesting surgery. Truly, he did all the right things within the limits of his belief system. Had she gone forward with the surgery, the surgical case review at the hospital would have approved his handling of the situation. And his treatment would have been effective. But effective or not, the surgery would have been unnecessary.

The gynecologist heard that Jane had gone to the other doctor. In the long run, the fact that Jane quit bleeding did not impress him. With an open invitation to learn something about the interaction between the mind and the body, he remains locked into his own belief system.

A metaphysical or eclectic approach to illness can mesh quite comfortably with what is considered standard practice. Certainly, the two approaches are different both in the model of disease development and in treatment, but they are not in hopeless conflict as we are so often led to believe. The comprehensive approach concerns itself more with the feelings, attitudes, beliefs, fears, convictions, goals, and aspirations of the patient. These are the elements that contribute to illness and recovery through the mind-body connection. For this reason, an eclectic physician is not limited to standard therapy when it proves ineffective.

If the body were not a construction of the psyche, then all approaches other than allopathy would amount only to so much mumbo jumbo. The fact that an inclusive approach to the maintenance of health and the treatment of disease is effective confirms the truth of this strategy. While the conventional doctor is writing a prescription for the latest pharmaceutical triumph, he is rarely aware that it is the patient's belief system that ultimately maintains her health or contributes to the onset of her illness. We may work in a technical and scientific world of physics, chemistry, tests, rules, and laws, but we live in a spiritual one.

CHAPTER NINE

ATTENDING YOUR BODY
NUTRITION

THERE ARE DOZENS of excellent books on nutrition that contain far more detailed information about food than I could possibly give here. I would not attempt to reproduce their work even if I could. Rather, I will give you some insights concerning how to care for your body, and information about nutrition that other books often omit.

Concern about your health and a desire to live a long, diseasefree life will accomplish little if you do not take care of your physical being. Intent alone will not prevent you from suffering the effects of malnutrition if you do not obtain the nutrients your body needs for growth and repair. We know we are constantly replacing our bodies and that without the proper nutrients in the right amounts and at the right time, it is impossible to perform this task efficiently, if at all. Over forty specific nutritional elements are required for life and health. These include essential proteins called amino acids, carbohydrates, various fatty acids found in fat and oil, minerals, vitamins, fiber, and water. Unless we manage to get all these nutrients on a more or less regular basis, we develop deficiency diseases, some of them deadly. Your body depends upon your eating properly; your cells can't send out to the corner deli for whatever your diet lacks.

A number of myths about nutrition seem embedded in the thinking of most doctors and of the public. First, we tend to believe that eating a balanced diet makes additional vitamins and minerals unnecessary. I would venture to say that *nobody* eats a balanced diet, at least not consistently. This fact was borne out by a study done about thirty years ago by a U.S. Senate task force investigating malnutrition in the United States. But over the years since, Americans have not improved their eating habits, and there is some indication that they have even worsened. Far too often, for instance, people either skip breakfast altogether or eat something quick and sweet. For too many, breakfast consists of coffee and a Danish during the midmorning break. Lunches are no less hectic. Most working people are allowed thirty minutes – time for a sandwich and coffee or a burger, fries, and a cola. And sitting down to a relaxed evening meal is often little more than a wish. Both parents are likely to work – sometimes on different schedules – and the kids are often too busy with their own activities to do much more than grab a bite on the run.

The "recommended daily requirements" also generate misconceptions. The new labeling system includes these amounts printed on every packaged food item. It's important to understand that these recommendations have little to do with *good* nutrition. The amounts listed for the various nutrients will do little more than prevent the average person from developing some nutritional deficiency disease. Not quite having scurvy or beriberi is a far cry from being ideally nourished. The trouble is that no one really knows the amount of any nutrient required for ideal nutrition. We don't even know how to measure ideal nutrition. If the recommended daily requirement is all they receive, most people will be truly undernourished. Animal studies have shown that, even among identical quadruplets, there are vast differences in the amount of various nutrients required by individuals. What we know is that in nature most living creatures, plant or animal, are skirting the edges of malnutrition most of the time. Food may be plentiful for a period of time and then hardly available. To be healthy, we must go far beyond any "recommended daily requirement."

Beyond this, most people are sorely mistaken about the levels of nutrients in the foods we eat. The amounts reported in books on nutrition are obtained through analysis of fresh, raw food that is garden ripened. No allowance is made for the nutrients destroyed by cooking, canning, freezing, and storage other than to state that there is "some loss." The foodstuffs available to the consumer, even the fresh ones, are not garden ripened. If the truck farmers waited to harvest until the vegetables and fruit were ripe, their produce would be spoiled long before it reached the market. I know of some cases of scurvy in people who were eating fresh oranges and grapefruit every day. This totally puzzled their doctors until the fruit was tested. The store-bought citrus was found to be virtually lacking in vitamin C. It seems that vitamin C does not form in the fruit until the end stages of ripening on the tree. Who among us has had the privilege of eating a tree-ripened orange? What is true for vitamin C holds true for many other nutrients.

The U.S. Food and Drug Administration (FDA), backed by Congress and the food industry, perpetuates the idea that taking vitamins is uncalled for and sometimes dangerous. Unfortunately, all too many medical doctors still echo this misinformation. I was appalled when I joined the Bellaire clinic to find that the obstetrician and pediatricians were not prescribing vitamins for their patients. Since nearly all their patients were to some degree obese, the doctors concluded they were "getting enough." They ignored the fact that in our patient population in the Ohio valley, the major sources of calories were pasta, soft drinks, potato chips, and snack cakes and an occasional piece of lunch meat. Most of the women and children were indeed obese, but they were also malnourished, and if one knew what to look for, many showed obvious signs of vitamin deficiency diseases.

Some years later, the obstetrician finally began giving the pregnant women iron, but only after the clinic was surveyed by a team from the Centers for Disease Control. Rarely did the pediatricians prescribe vitamins unless a child was thin and lacked an appetite.

The idea that vitamins are dangerous began when the members of Admiral Perry's expedition were trying to reach the North Pole and became lost, separated from their supplies. With what they thought was luck, they shot a polar bear. Knowing that liver contains many nutrients, they gorged on polar bear liver. What they did not know was that polar bear liver contains the highest concentration of vitamin A to be found anywhere. Vitamin A, being fat soluble, is not readily eliminated. It is estimated that they consumed several million units of vitamin A, resulting in severe toxicity, and some of them died.

Then, when vitamin D was found to prevent rickets, many doctors reasoned that it would also be effective in treating arthritis. But vitamin D is also fat soluble and is not quickly eliminated from the body. Massive doses of vitamin D did not help patients' arthritis but did cause many of them to develop massive calcium deposits throughout their bodies. At toxic levels, vitamin D calcified their tendons, ligaments, blood vessels, eyeballs, and kidneys. Again, some patients died or were rendered blind. As a result, medical doctors pronounced that vitamins were dangerous – and they were, when prescribed at these toxic levels.

To maintain your health, you must understand that taking vitamins is safe. You'd have to go way out of your way to do yourself any harm with vitamins. Vitamin A can be taken in doses as high as 10,000 to 15,000 units daily. Vitamin D is perfectly safe in amounts up to 800 units daily, except in rare instances. It is true that vitamin D is formed in your skin by sunlight affecting your skin oils, but the amount is negligible. Furthermore, if you bathe daily, the skin oils are not present on the surface of your body to be converted to vitamin D.

Vitamin E, a fat-soluble vitamin, can be taken in doses as high as 10,000 units. It is an important antioxidant and helps protect your body from chemical fragments called free radicals that can do considerable damage to cells and are thought to contribute to the aging process.

All other vitamins are water soluble and nontoxic. Doctors often say it is pointless to take these in large amounts, for they are immediately eliminated from the body. If this were a valid reason, then it would be pointless to give large doses of penicillin to treat infections, for it's known that penicillin is excreted in a matter of hours. The value in giving large doses of some substances is that it bathes the tissues with high concentrations of the medicine even though the body doesn't retain it for extended periods of time. The same is true for vitamins.

All warm-blooded animals manufacture vitamin C in their livers as a by-product of glucose metabolism. Cold-blooded animals produce vitamin C in much smaller amounts in their kidneys. The only animals that do not produce vitamin C are humans, primates, guinea pigs, a fruit-eating bat in India, and a fruit-eating warbler in Asia. It turns out that the average vitamin C production among all the other animals is 200 milligrams for every kilogram of body weight every twenty-four hours. To simplify, let's say they produce 100 milligrams for every pound of body weight a day. This means that a tapir or a wildebeest that weighs 150 pounds would be making 15,000 milligrams of vitamin C every day. Since no healthy biological system overproduces in a wasteful manner, we can conclude that these creatures *require* these amounts for proper health. And the ridiculous amount recommended by the FDA for an adult human is a meager 60 milligrams.

The discoverer of vitamin C, Albert Szent-Gyorgyi, who received the Nobel Prize for his work, said that instead of being sold in drugstores by the milligram, vitamin C should be sold in grocery stores by the pound. Some years previously he had developed pneumonia and was dying despite receiving the best medical care. Thinking about his plight, he realized he was exhibiting many of the same symptoms as his laboratory animals that had scurvy. He had always taken 1,000 milligrams of vitamin C every day, but with the stress of his illness it was obviously not enough. He immediately increased his intake to 8,000 milligrams, and within three days he was well and back working in his laboratory.

Szent-Gyorgyi believed that if he had not increased his vitamin C intake he would have died. He was certain that his death certificate would have listed the cause of death as pneumonia, when in reality it would have been scurvy, with the pneumonia merely being an opportunistic infection.

Besides preventing scurvy, among other things vitamin C is necessary for normal white blood cell functioning and the formation of scars. There is also very strong evidence that large doses kill viruses and assist body defenses against cancerous growths.

In the previous chapter, I wrote about Ted, who was treated for his impending heart attack by the nutritionist who put him on a low-salt diet. Overconsumption of table salt is one of the major nutritional problems today. I realize that we no longer hear much about salt. The present fad is to eliminate fat and carbohydrates from the diet. Nevertheless, the high-sodium diet most Americans consume is the cornerstone for the development of virtually all arteriosclerotic cardiovascular diseases. This list includes high blood pressure, heart attacks, hardening of the arteries, strokes, arteriosclerotic gangrene of the legs, and heart failure.

Sodium found in table salt and other food additives has a negative impact on health because of its effect on the metabolism of heart muscle cells and the smooth muscle cells in the arterial walls. While it is common practice for doctors to prescribe low-salt diets, rarely do they adequately stress the importance of the diet for all of us, nor do they reduce the sodium intake enough for total effectiveness.

Some years ago, I went to a medical meeting with over four hundred internists. A speaker from the Mayo clinic gave a paper on the treatment of high blood pressure. He began by listing the steps in the treatment of hypertension. The first step, he said, was for the doctor to throwaway his prescription pad. All the doctors gasped. The second step was to put the patient on a very low salt diet. He suggested something in the range of 750 to 1,000 milligrams of sodium. Most of us eat at least 3,500 milligrams of sodium daily, and some people consume as much as 20,000 milligrams. Then, after a couple of weeks, the speaker advised, check the patient's blood pressure. If it is not down, test the daily urinary output for sodium to see whether the patient is following the diet. If not, the patient should be urged to follow the recommendation. Then, he said, and only as a last resort, when the diet is unsuccessful, write a prescription for one or more of the many excellent drugs on the market. He didn't discuss the drugs, for he considered them all of secondary importance. Instead, he continued to speak to the value of reducing sodium in the diet.

We all need to guard against becoming caught up in every nutritional fad that comes along. Every week or two some science story in the news cautions us concerning one illness or another said to be caused or worsened by something we eat. The cholesterol scare started about fifty years ago when doctors learned that the fatty plaques in arteries contain cholesterol compounds. Everyone was warned not to eat eggs and other foods that contained cholesterol. Low-cholesterol diets are somewhat effective in lowering the cholesterol, but only if they are also low in saturated fat. In addition, doctors did not take into account that cholesterol is a huge molecule and is not directly absorbed by the intestine into the bloodstream. Cholesterol is digested into smaller molecular fragments before it is absorbed by the gut. Saturated fats raise cholesterol levels in the body because they stimulate the liver to produce excess cholesterol.

I had heard this for years when attending lectures on nutrition, and some time ago I decided to test the idea myself. I had many patients on low-cholesterol and low-saturated-fat diets. With their permission, I had my ten most faithful patients continue to avoid the saturated fats but instructed them to eat two eggs for breakfast every day. After two weeks, I had their cholesterol levels checked. The addition of two eggs to their diet did not raise their blood cholesterol one iota.

But we must be careful in avoiding fats. Certainly saturated fats are a problem, but the body needs certain fats for good nutrition. These are found in vegetable, olive, canola, and fish oil. Meat fat and the hard, white, solid cooking fats that don't melt on the shelf are high in saturated fat, and these cause the body to respond by making cholesterol. Pork and chicken fat, by the way, contain far less saturated fat than does the fat found in beef and lamb. Reducing our meat intake is helpful because it lowers the risk of atherosclerosis as well as wear and tear on our kidneys, which have to excrete the waste products of metabolized protein.

One nutrient the public never hears about is magnesium, which is essential in muscle and nerve metabolism. Americans are all deficient in magnesium, except perhaps people in those cultures that eat large quantities of beans and the old folks who take their milk of magnesia every night before going to bed. As Mildred Selig found almost thirty years ago, serum magnesium levels do not properly reflect deficiencies, because magnesium, like potassium, moves out of the cells into the blood in order to maintain critical levels in the serum. Thus, long before the blood levels fall, the cells of the body have been dangerously depleted of both magnesium and potassium. Magnesium and potassium deficiencies are two of the factors that make Americans prone to heart attacks. And magnesium deficiency is the cause of most "pulled muscles" seen in athletes as well as leg cramps experienced at night.

The following cases illustrate the importance of good overall nutrition.

I recall a patient who was presented to the hospital staff as a case study. Semicomatose, she was wheeled into the conference room for us to see. The lady had been admitted through the emergency room with a ruptured peptic ulcer. In this condition, the ulcer actually eats a hole through the intestinal wall and gut contents spill out into the abdomen. It is extremely serious and often fatal if surgery or some type of intervention is not performed promptly. On admission, the patient gave a history of smoking two packs of cigarettes a day and drinking a six-pack of soda pop daily. Cookies, potato chips, crackers, and an occasional piece of lunch meat rounded out her diet. She was immediately taken to surgery and the ruptured ulcer was repaired.

Following surgery, she did not do well. She developed an ileus, a condition in which the intestine ceases to function normally to carry fluids and gas. Her abdomen became very distended, and one week after her surgery, her wound fell apart and had to be resutured. Her intestinal tract continued to remain nonfunctional. At the time she was presented to the staff, it had been over three weeks since her original surgery. The woman still had a stomach tube and was being given intravenous fluids. Earlier, she had developed pneumonia and was now in a semicoma, mumbling incoherently to herself and picking at her blankets and sheets. Laboratory tests and X-rays were of no help in determining the cause of her complications and the intestinal ileus.

Looking at the woman, I was stunned at what I saw. She had numerous bruises where the nurses had taken hold of her to turn her in bed. In spite of adequate fluid in her system, her skin lacked resiliency. Her abdomen was still swollen and doughy on palpation. She looked horrible and probably would have told us that she felt worse if she could have spoken coherently. She seemed to me to present a clear picture of severe malnutrition and had the complications to prove it. In the first place, prior to the rupture of her ulcer, she had been getting the bulk of her calories from soda pop, chips, and cookies. Thus far, three weeks into treatment, she had not had a single meal in the hospital. From the history alone I knew that she was deficient in protein and all the vitamins and minerals. Without adequate magnesium and vitamin B6, the brain, nerves, and muscles, including the muscles in the intestinal wall, cannot work properly. This alone could account for her intestinal ileus, her confusion, and her coma. Wounds do not heal without vitamin C, folic acid, and zinc. Cell division is dependent on many things, including folic acid. If nothing else, the bruises hinted at a vitamin C deficiency, and it is known that without adequate vitamin C, infections are a common occurrence. Most people with scurvy die of infections of one form or another. These were but a few of my observations.

Her doctor had been giving her some multivitamins in the intravenous feedings, but the amount was grossly inadequate for normal nutrition, much less for treating an individual who had not been eating well and was under tremendous physiologic stress. Moreover, the vitamin supplement did not contain folic acid. When it came time for comments, I told the staff that I felt her basic problem was severe malnutrition. They laughed uproariously, insisting that her case was one of a ruptured peptic ulcer complicated by postoperative pneumonia and disruption of the wound. I agreed that the ruptured ulcer had brought her to the hospital, but that had been taken care of the night of admission. The pneumonia had been adequately treated with antibiotics and her belly resutured. I insisted they now had a woman dying of malnutrition. But they continued to laugh. Several days later, her doctor approached me and asked what supplements I would prescribe. I recited a long list of large doses of vitamins and minerals. He took some of my advice but did not give nearly the amount required to turn the tide quickly. Slowly, the patient began to improve, but it took another two months for her to become sufficiently well to leave the hospital.

One day, a young man was literally carried into my office by his parents. He was too weak to walk on his own. He had been living in a commune outside Denver and had contracted hepatitis. He was so jaundiced that his skin was orange. His liver was hugely enlarged, and the liver function tests were off the charts. He was able to eat and take fluids, so there was no point in placing him in the hospital. The parents asked if there was any treatment that might facilitate his recovery. I explained that hepatitis is a viral disease and therefore antibiotics were of no value. I added that many veterinarians had been curing distemper in puppies with large amounts of vitamin C for years. I suggested he take as much vitamin C as he could tolerate. He started on a dose of 50,000 milligrams a day. The next day the parents called, saying that he had developed diarrhea. At my suggestion, he cut back on the dosage and finally settled on 26,000 milligrams. One week later the young man walked into my office. His jaundice was gone and his liver was no longer enlarged. The tests were all back to normal except for a minimal elevation of his alkaline phosphatase.

Furthermore, he felt so well that, for the previous two days, he had been in the woods with his father using a chain saw and an ax to cut firewood. Under the more standard treatments, hepatitis just does not recover that fast. There's no doubt in my mind that the vitamin C made the difference.

People often bring in more problems than their initially stated reason for consulting a doctor. One man I treated had advanced hardening of the arteries in his legs, resulting in terrible circulation. At the time I saw him, surgical removal of certain nerve ganglia that controlled vascular tone in the leg vessels was an accepted treatment. He had consulted a surgeon, who performed the operation, but six days following the surgery, his incision had fallen apart, and he required a second operation to repair the wound disruption. The man felt he had not been sewn up properly the first time.

I had assisted in the original surgery and did, in fact, resuture his wound, because his surgeon was ill and unable to perform the operation. I was not surprised that the man eviscerated. He smoked heavily and had emphysema and a bad cough. Furthermore, his nutrition was terrible. The stitches had not given way; the tissues had simply fallen apart as a result of the malnutrition and the constant coughing. Certainly, the man had a circulation problem, but he entered the hospital suffering from malnutrition and chronic obstructive lung disease as well.

This case demonstrates the importance of assessing the entire patient. The surgeon should have recognized that the man was poorly nourished and needed high doses of multivitamins and minerals before he was scheduled for surgery. The patient's circulation problem posed no emergency so severe that the surgery could not have been scheduled for two or three weeks later. But specialists, as a group, have a tendency to evaluate their patients through the narrowed view of their training. And their training rarely includes much about nutrition.

Taking care of your body also entails getting exercise of one kind or another. Exercising until you look like a bodybuilder is not the key to good health. Neither is running mile after mile every day. Studies have shown that marathon runners are no more protected from heart attacks than people who do not exercise at all. In addition, jogging produces impact injuries to the feet, ankles, and knees. Running also causes the abdominal muscles to become weak, and this tends to produce hyperextension of the lumbar spine, resulting in backaches. All the early studies concerning the beneficial effects of exercise on cardiovascular fitness were done on people who *walked.* When those studies became public, the sports enthusiasts and those who manufacture sporting equipment promoted the idea that if walking was good, jogging and running would be better. They aren't. And in addition to its being a low-impact exercise, walking has an added benefit. It allows us to visit with a companion and hear the birds and the breeze in the trees. Joggers are more apt to be hearing only their own gasps for breath.

If you are to be healthy, my advice is to eat as balanced a meal as possible most of the time. Eat less protein and increase your intake of vegetables and fruit. Take time to enjoy what you eat, and if this includes having a glass of wine with the evening meal, so be it. Try to avoid eating saturated fats, salt, and foods known to contain chemicals, herbicides, and pesticides. And take a walk at least four or five times a week.

After doing all this, you still need to take nutritional supplements. Take a therapeutic multivitamin-mineral supplement once daily. In addition to that, take a *minimum* of 1,000 milligrams of vitamin C twice a day. Add to this 400 to 800 units of vitamin E and a couple of 250 milligram tablets of magnesium oxide. If you do not or cannot eat milk products without developing gas from the lactose, take about 1,500 milligrams of calcium or use lactose free milk. Many antacid medicines contain calcium carbonate and are far less costly than medicines that contain the same form of calcium.

If you're doing all that, you can worry a bit less about your weight. The Framingham study conducted at Harvard medical school showed a surprising thing about obesity. The investigators found that if the obesity did not contribute to the person's having high blood pressure or to the development of diabetes, and if the cholesterol level was not high, *it didn't seem to matter how much the person weighed!* If these factors were not involved, the study found, then there was no correlation between body weight and risk of a cardiovascular event. A cardiovascular event was defined as a heart attack, a stroke, hypertensive heart failure, or arteriosclerotic gangrene of the leg.

Of course, there are other health risks for the very obese. They have more accidents, backaches, and arthritis of the knees, and, if they are confined to bed for whatever reason, they have a greater risk of developing pneumonia. But your weight is simply not a good indicator of your overall health.

The entire purpose of eating is to give the body adequate amounts of calories, water, roughage, protein, carbohydrates, fats, and minerals to build new cells and repair damaged ones. Vitamins act as catalysts (facilitators) to help the cells assimilate and process the food. No vitamin pill will enable you to eat junk food every day and still receive good nutrition. You need to eat the best diet you can *and* take the vitamin-mineral supplement. Just because I have stressed that many foods do not contain the amount of vitamins we are led to believe, does not mean that the foods are completely lacking in nutrition. Minerals, protein, carbohydrates, fats, and some vitamins survive canning, cooking, and so on. So eat the best balanced diet you can.

The important thing to remember is that you are meant to enjoy life. Eating is one of life's pleasures. You will not drop dead tomorrow if you occasionally indulge in a hamburger and fries at your local fast food restaurant. You will do far more harm to yourself if you spend your time worrying about everything you eat, convinced that lurking within every morsel is some nameless danger against which you have yet to be warned.

If you add good nutrition to your positive intent to be healthy, you will aid your bioconsciousness in its ability to repair damage, renew itself, and recover from disease.

CHAPTER TEN

MIRACULOUS HEALING

HOW IT WORKS

C ERTAINLY, IN EVERY DISCUSSION of spontaneous or self-healing, sooner or later the subject of miracles arises. Miracles are considered to be extranormal events caused by some outside force or being. But the mechanisms producing such leaps into health and wholeness are precisely those that have been discussed in the previous chapters.

Everyone is familiar with the existence of religious shrines at which miracles are said to occur. All organized religions have them. We of the Western world are more familiar with the ones associated with the Roman Catholic church, which are scattered all over the globe. And now that religious programs are seen regularly on television, we are treated to spectacles of healing on a more or less regular basis. We can no longer dismiss all these cures as hoaxes set up by insincere preachers with accomplices who are actors or shills. The shrines at Lourdes and the cathedrals in Quebec have too many crutches and built-up shoes left hanging at the altar to allow dismissal of spiritual healings. But science and common sense tell us that a short leg does not suddenly become longer. Diabetes does not just go away. A deaf person does not immediately regain her hearing just because some preacher prays, pushes her in the forehead, and shouts, "Woo!" So what are we to believe? Is something else going on that the scientific world has yet to discover or admit?

First of all, let's admit that many "cures" are not easily documented. Whether I have pain or not is a purely subjective experience. I can tell you that my back is hurting, but who else can know? Even physicians are hard-pressed at times to tell whether their patients are malingering or are really ill or in pain.

We do know that most spontaneous healings are the effects highly charged experiences in which a number of things happen. Take, for example, the individual who goes to an evangelist's prayer meeting with great expectations of being healed of his chronic back injury. Knowing ahead of time that he will attend the meeting, he has psychologically worked himself up to expect a cure and has prepared himself for something miraculous. In the fervor of the meeting and the company of a highly charged, charismatic preacher, he actually does feel better, *and believes it in his heart.* It is an established phenomenon that, when our attention is directed elsewhere, many aches and pains go unnoticed. This is a common occurrence in sports, when severe injuries often go undetected until after the game. Add to this that, in the presence of his friends and neighbors, the sufferer at the prayer meeting is reluctant to say that he was *not* cured, if for no other reason than that he does not wish to appear lacking in faith. In the euphoria of the event and with the pain temporarily gone, even his range of motion may become normal. Not often is there any physical alteration in the body that limits motion. Usually it is pain and fear of doing damage to oneself that limit the ability to move. Lacking pain, and with the belief that his infirmity is cured, the believer's range of motion may well return to normal. Such a "spiritual" event is not unlike waking hypnosis, in which all sorts of suggestions may be given and accepted by the subject.

The proof of the cure lies in its permanence. If the symptoms begin to recur in the next few hours or days, the individual is likely to be filled with guilt, for his faith in God is on the line. He might perceive himself as having been unworthy of a real cure. Often he will be unwilling to admit the truth even to himself. Failure to obtain a miracle is often very damaging to one's sense of self-worth.

But real cures do occur. Approximately 3 or 4 percent of miraculous cures are true, permanent healings. They are the result of one of two things, or a combination: a shift of probabilities or a dramatic and newly adopted belief system. Let us discuss probability shifts first. To understand probability shifts you will have to think back to our discussion of Framework II, where everything exists at once in a network of probability.

To understand the temporal reality in which we live, it will be helpful to visualize energy lines going out in all directions from every moment. Think of these energy lines as shadows of reality, potential events waiting to be actualized. Now, remember our discussion about physicists speaking of these potentials as "the sum over histories" and their attempt to explain why particles act as they do. The particles, experiments have revealed, appear to be in communication with physicists and to know their intent. In apparent response to that intent, the particles choose to energize one probability among the infinite possibilities and thereby do what the physicists want. In the same manner and at every moment, you choose certain actions on the basis of your beliefs about yourself, the Universe, your culture, and your past experiences. Then you generate a choice to energize certain probabilities in Framework II and make them a part of your temporal reality, Framework I.

All of the potential paths relating to your life – these shadows of unrealized probabilities – have a very real existence. Existing along in parallel dimensions are other dimensions of yourself, which are known as probable selves, living and exercising other potential choices.

This network of potential, unrealized events represents one explanation of relative time. Relative time can be visualized as a vast lacework of interplaying energy in which every conceivable probability of every probable event is imprinted upon the network of possibility. Traversing the network, we energize the paths of our choice as we go along. Thus, it can be stated that everything happens at once, since every possibility always exists, whether our actions have chosen it or not.

From the vantage point of Framework II, your life appears as a syncytium of interactions in which your probable selves act and react, exchanging thoughts, behaviors, and activities in the vast labyrinthine system of relative time.

An example may make all this more clear. Assume that at one time you strongly considered marrying your high school sweetheart. Because of choices made by both of you, her life drifted from yours and you both married different people. As a youth, you had been intensely interested in art but confined your interest to the pleasure of looking at photographs of artworks. In high school, you had a gift for talking with people, and your friends used to come to you with their problems. You seriously considered going to college and being a psychologist but, because of the time involved and your need to make a living, you chose to become a plumber. These probabilities will be sufficient to illustrate the process.

In the terms we're using here, you have a probable self who married your sweetheart, another who became an artist, and a third who went to college and majored in psychology.

But because of the intense focus in the temporal reality of Framework I, you are unaware of these probable selves. One day, while redecorating the office in your plumbing business, the thought occurs to you that a mural might be nice and that maybe you'll just try doing it yourself. You find yourself painting beautifully, drawing upon the probable self that did pursue the probability of becoming an artist. At times, you find yourself thinking about your old love and it almost seems as if you did marry her. Despite being happily married to your wife, you continue to feel very close to your old sweetheart, though you've not seen or heard from her in twenty years. People come into your office just to talk with you because you continue to have an uncanny, intuitive knowledge about people and have genuinely helped many of your customers and friends who are troubled. They may even say that you're more help than their doctor or psychiatrist. These unexplained talents and feelings are subtle exchanges of talents, knowledge, and love from your probable selves.

Seen from the constraints of this temporal reality, you are a plumber and nothing more. Being unaware of probable selves, you may puzzle over your feelings about your old girlfriend, your unexplained talent for painting, and your flair for talking to people about their troubles, but this is as far as it goes. Each probable self is as real as you are. To them, you are a probable self who became a plumbing contractor. The probable self who is the artist might just have a knack for repairing his own plumbing.

Choosing a probability to actualize involves other things' health, for example. Picture yourself hiking in the mountains. You come to a very dangerous place where a missed step could result in a bad fall. A number of probable events focus upon this point in time. You may proceed along without difficulty. You may fall and sustain a broken arm and be disabled thereafter. You may fall and be killed. You might even have

179

taken a different turn and not been confronted with the choices. Assume you were not paying attention and chose the probability that led to the broken arm. If you were able to shift probabilities, your broken arm could be avoided by jumping from the probability in which you fell to the one that led to an uneventful, pleasant hike through the mountains, or to one in which you did not go hiking at all. If a probability shift were to occur, then you would not have fallen, no fracture would have ensued, and you would have proceeded with a life in which you had never been hurt.

Incident after incident in our world serves as evidence that such a probability shift is at times attainable. Neither of the following examples involves healing, but the principle of action involved is the same. And they do constitute "miracles."

I know a young couple who were driving over the mountains in New Mexico a few winters ago. The roads were snowy and quite treacherous. On the particular stretch of secondary highway they were traveling along, there was no guardrail, only a fairly wide shoulder. They were going downhill and came to a sharp curve that was especially icy. Their car lost traction and, instead of following the curve, it began to skid straight toward the cliff's edge. The man did his best to control the skid, but the car seemed to pick up speed as it slid. Both he and his wife looked in horror at the edge of the shoulder as their car left the highway and, with no sign of slowing, headed for the hundred-foot drop. An instant before his car reached the lip of the canyon, he shouted, "NO!" It was a silent scream – just to himself and the Universe. Suddenly, there was a sort of jerk within their bodies, a split second of disorientation, and then they found their car some twenty feet from where it had been a moment before, in the proper lane on the highway, completely under control, going around the curve with no evidence of skidding or any steering problem. Both the man and his wife experienced the same thing. This is a perfect example of jumping from one probability, in which they slid off the cliff, into another, in which a skid did not occur.

It was like a quantum jump that takes place in subatomic physics. When electrons jump from one orbit to another, they cannot be found in the "between" state. They are in one orbit or the other, and physicists never find them starting to leave, or arriving, or halfway between the orbits. So it was with my friends in the skidding car. One moment they were literally a few inches from the edge of the drop-off, and then, instantaneously, they were some twenty feet away, back on the road, proceeding normally around the curve. They happened to be alone on that small stretch of the highway, but if people in another car had chanced to see the event, they might have described it this way: "Boy, did you see that car? I thought it was skidding off the road, but I guess my eyes were playing tricks on me. I'd better get a cup of coffee." Unless we know about jumping probabilities, we are completely unaware of the phenomenon even when we see it happen.

A somewhat similar event happened in my own life. During the Korean War, I was stationed at Camp Lejeune with the Second Marine Division as a battalion surgeon. We were making a practice landing in very rough weather; the ocean swells were a good sixteen feet high. We were debarking from the troop ship, going down cargo nets into the landing craft. The landing boats were slamming against the side of the ship with each swell, making the transfer very dangerous. If the cargo net was not kept inside the landing craft, a person descending the net could find himself crushed between the landing craft and the ship as they came smashing together with the next swell. One instant a man would be almost to the deck of the landing craft and the next instant he would be six or eight feet above the side of the boat as the swell dropped away.

As I was descending the net, I looked down and saw that my corpsmen were doing their job keeping the net inside the landing craft. I hurried down and suddenly realized I was between the ship and the landing craft, which was high above me. I was a good ten feet below the craft, almost in the water. I experienced a split second of panic in which I was certain I was going to be crushed, followed by a clear belief that I was all right. At the same instant I found myself stepping off the net into the boat. I asked my chief how I had made it and he couldn't give me an answer. He mumbled something about being lucky. At the time, I knew nothing of probability shifts, but I am quite certain that was what kept me from severe injury or death. In that moment, I changed probabilities to end up in the boat rather than crushed between the ships.

In a spontaneous healing, the probability shift is sudden and dramatic, as it was with my friends in the skidding car and with me on the cargo net. Often, when a healing occurs, there will be a second or two of confusion or disorientation in which the beneficiary's perception is blurred. When her mind clears, she will realize something has happened. She no longer finds herself crippled or ill. She no longer has the infirmity that existed in the other line of probability.

I'm convinced that probability shifts are not rare occurrences. They are only rarely understood and recognized. However, in recent years, these types of healing events have been rarely seen, even in churches. This is because our false sense of sophistication and our belief in science rather than in faith literally blocks probability shifts.

A few years ago, I was discussing probability shifts with an acquaintance who listened intently and then related this experience. In the town where he lives, he is a member of the local emergency squad. One day the squad was called to an auto accident in which a young girl had been badly injured. They rushed the unconscious, bleeding girl to the local hospital, where it was found that she was suffering from a severe head injury and a skull fracture. In addition, she had major fractures of an arm and a leg. The local hospital was not equipped to treat such a severe head injury, so they took X-rays, stabilized her, splinted the fractures, and arranged for immediate air transport to a large hospital in Denver. The local doctor called ahead with information about the condition of the girl so the emergency room in Denver could begin treatment immediately.

In the meantime, word went out among the townspeople of the child's desperate condition. Without any prior arrangement, members of the girl's church contacted one another, and within half an hour, some one hundred and fifty people were praying for her. My friend said that the response was spontaneous and intense. In the meantime, the helicopter arrived, loaded the girl, and headed for the Denver hospital, where she was whisked from the landing pad to the emergency room.

A short time later the doctor in Denver called the doctor in the small town wanting to know what all the fuss was about. The girl, it seems, had no cuts, no head injury, no skull fracture, and no broken bones in her arm or leg. In Denver, they had taken X rays and compared them with the ones taken at the local hospital about an hour previously. The new ones revealed no injuries. Their explanation was that somehow the X rays had been mislabeled by the local hospital and were of some other patient. The doctor in Denver did not admit the girl but sent her home, for he could find nothing wrong with her.

Unequivocating, focused intent can create healings without the addition of probability shifts. These events are explained on the basis that it is mind that creates matter. You will recall the earlier discussion about consciousness-units and their ability to organize matter about them. It was explained that the consciousness, awareness, memory, communication, intent, creativity and precognition of the consciousness-units give matter its qualities of life. You will recall that the consciousness-units create an energy pattern upon which matter forms. When we are injured or ill, the energy pattern is not altered. If you have a leg amputated, the energy pattern of the missing leg does not go away but remains forever.

The phenomenon in which a dramatic shift in belief system produces physical changes is clearly demonstrated in some cases of multiple personalities. It has been documented that when multiple personalities have their personality fragments rigidly compartmentalized, the personalities do not necessarily have the same illnesses. In one documented case, one personality was diabetic and required rather large doses of insulin, and the other personality was not diabetic at all. In another instance, one personality had normal vision without glasses, whereas the other personality was very nearsighted and required an exceedingly strong correction to see anything at all. In yet another case, one personality was terribly allergic to tomatoes and broke out in a rash in his mouth and around his face every time he ate even a small piece of tomato. An alternate personality had no such allergy and was, in fact, fond of Italian food covered with various tomato sauces. This sort of thing is possible because the personality (the mind) always determines our physical status. In the above cases, the "other" personalities did not wish to be nearsighted, diabetic, or allergic to tomatoes, so their bodies conformed to their intense, unspoken belief that they were normal. If a person with multiple personalities can alter his vision, allergies, or illnesses as he quickly shifts from one personality to another, there is nothing to prevent a patient who is ill from utilizing his intent to be well by doing the same thing.

When an evangelist effects a healing, the believer may suddenly and unequivocally adopt a new belief system concerning her illness or disability. We speak of this phenomenon as a miracle. In a very real sense, when you do this, you are doing exactly what the multiple personality patient does. What you need to comprehend is that it is not necessary to go to a healer of any sort, medical, religious, or otherwise, to accomplish this task. All that is required on your part is unwavering belief that it can be done and an unequivocally focused intent to be whole. The bioconsciousness will do the rest.

When I first started practice, a high school senior who was a patient of mine developed a very rare ovarian cancer. By the time she consulted me, it had spread throughout her body. Her abdomen was so full of tumor and fluid that she appeared to be seven or eight months pregnant. Her lungs contained huge masses of tumor as well. I operated on her, obtained a biopsy of the tumor, and sewed her up. There was no treatment at that time for her type of cancer. This was in April.

A week after the surgery, I repeated the X ray of her chest and the tumors were gone! Neither had the fluid reaccumulated in her abdomen. The radiologist said that if he had not seen it himself, he would have thought the dates on the X rays had gotten mixed up.

The girl returned to school, made up her lost time, and graduated with her class. That fall, she worked in a department store earning money to buy her brother and parents Christmas presents. All the while, she remained healthy and apparently tumor free. But after Christmas she began to develop signs of her cancer again. I was forced repeatedly to tap her lungs and abdomen and remove huge quantities of fluid filled with cancerous cells to make her more comfortable and allow her to breathe.

On Easter Sunday, she got out of bed, dressed in her finest Easter clothes, and went to church. That afternoon about 2 P.M., her father called, saying that his daughter wanted to be admitted to the hospital. I admitted her about 3 P.M. She said, "Gee, Dr. Bonnett, dying of cancer isn't so painful. It's just miserable. Could you give me a shot so I can get some sleep?

I'm so tired." I complied with her wish, stayed with her until the medicine took effect, and then left. About an hour later, the hospital called to say that she was dead.

Her father was a minister, and she had missed Easter services the year before because of her surgery. I learned that when she was diagnosed with cancer, she made a deal with God. She asked God to allow her to live until after the next Easter Sunday so that she could hear her father give one more Easter sermon. That is what she got. Had I known then what I know now, I might have shown her that if she could make her cancer go away for nine months, there was the possibility that she could make it disappear for a longer time or completely.

Three years ago, a friend of mine developed cancer of the lung. Jerry underwent all the usual medical procedures, such as radiation therapy, and even received some experimental drugs. At the same time, he was working with Greg Satre, who was instructing him in various methods of visualization and urging him to focus his intent upon the cancer going away and the cells returning to their normal pattern of growth. Jerry would meditate on the X-ray table and spiritual entities appeared to him. He told me that they imparted a great deal of metaphysical information and specific directions to him concerning his meditation and the healing of his cancer. These visualizations were highly successful and, within several months, Jerry was pronounced by his doctors to be tumor free.

Things seemed to be going well until he suddenly had a recurrence of his cancer and, within a month, died on Christmas Day. Greg and I were completely puzzled by this turn of events until after the funeral, when we spoke with his wife. She informed us that Jerry had made a deal with the Universe asking for one more year, or until he had time to get some property sold and all his financial deals settled. He completed his final business just one month before he died. Our friend was not religious in the classical sense, but his intent to have his tumor regress, allowing him time to organize his business affairs, followed the same mechanism as religious healings in which focused intent is used. In *The Secret Science Behind the Miracles,* Max Freedom Long provides a detailed discussion of the mechanism behind the miracle cures performed by Polynesian priests. They talk of the shadowy body that remains intact and the ability of their "magic" to cause matter to realign itself along the intact pattern of the shadowy body. Long writes of having witnessed events such as healing fractures and walking on hot lava flows without being burned.

In *Mutant Message Down Under,* Dr. Marlo Morgan describes watching a compound fracture of a shinbone heal on a walkabout with a group of Australian aborigines. It was a bad fracture, with several inches of broken bone protruding from a jagged tear. In the event Dr. Morgan witnessed, a man called Great Stone Hunter volunteered to have an accident arranged by the Universe. This was at the group's request, for they wished to demonstrate to the American doctor their ability to heal injuries and illnesses. Dr. Morgan stood beside the injured man while two other aborigines named Medicine Man and Female Healer performed the feat of instantly healing the fracture. They held the broken leg, passed their hands over it (but did not touch it) while chanting with the injured man, and suddenly, without pulling or traction of any kind, the broken bone slid back into the wound. They pushed the jagged edges of the torn skin together with their fingers, smeared the wound with decomposed menstrual blood, and the healing was complete. They explained that they had simply talked to the fractured bone, reminding it of its original pattern. The next day, the man continued the walkabout with no sign of having been injured.

Greg Satre has reported healings using the same psychic technique, which he worked out himself. I gave him a copy of

Long's book, and he was surprised that the explanation of the healing of a fracture was identical to what he had observed himself. He told me that he had once healed a fracture in a girl's foot. As he was watching the energy patterns, the broken bone seemed to go into an amorphous, nonaligned state and lost its configuration. Suddenly, he said, a second later, the bone reappeared completely healed. Immediately, the girl was able to walk and jump about with no discomfort whatsoever. The swelling and discoloration of the tissues about the fracture site were gone within a half hour. The next day, the healing event was confirmed by X ray. The film showed a healed fracture that appeared to be about six months old.

I said earlier that we age for many reasons, not the least of which is that we expect to age. If you determine that you are content at the age of forty and would like to have your body remain that way, to a large degree it is possible to do so, *providing your belief is intensely focused.* You can direct your intent to restructure your body continuously along the forty-year-old blueprint. One difficulty is that, no matter how intense your psychic focus and determination may be, society seems against you. All around you, you see your friends aging. They talk about being over the hill. Your children and spouse, commercials on television and advertisements in magazines, and numerous other factors reinforce the idea that you are getting older all the time. With each birthday you receive humorous cards depicting your becoming more senile by the minute. All these suggestions interfere with your focused intent.

We observe similar things happening to individuals who are ill when others, unwittingly or otherwise, hinder their intentions to be well. Even hospitals, which are supposed to be institutions of healing, are literally dens of misdirected intent. There the patient is surrounded by others who are ill and dying. The institutional emphasis is upon the tests and the treatment being ordered by the doctors. And the doctors, nurses, and visitors often make the most unsuitable statements to one who is attempting to get well. The attitude is one in which the patient is seen as a victim. I recall a time when my mother was ill. As she began to recover, friends would come to the house to call. In the course of conversation, they would ask her how she was feeling. When she indicated that she was getting better, I would hear them say things such as, "Now don't be too sure. My aunt thought she was getting better and she took a turn for the worse and died three days later." This sort of reaction on the part of others is why my friend who developed cancer of his colon told no one, not his mother, his children, or his closest friends. He knew that, regardless of their best wishes, their comments would be a distraction to his focused intent to cure himself.

There is yet another factor to consider: karma. Karma is an East Indian word meaning "fate". We often hear people say, "You don't die unless your number is up." Expressions such as these are nothing more than testimony to a belief in karma. In other chapters, I talk about there being no mistakes or errors. Illness and injury are windows to enlightenment and are planned at the psychological level of Framework II by the individuals themselves. If there is some karmic reason why the illness or infirmity is essential, no amount of medical, religious, or psychic intervention will be of any help. Failure to obtain a spiritual or psychic cure does not necessarily imply a lack of faith or that one is being punished for some sin, original or otherwise. What it does imply is that we all are subject to wiser plans and arrangements that take place in Framework II and with which we agree and comply.

Once the lesson is mastered, there are times when being disabled or chronically ill no longer serves any purpose. It has been said that the only purpose in suffering is to learn how not to suffer. During these times, people get well spontaneously through their focused intent to heal themselves or through a probability shift. However, as I indicated earlier, one must be willing to surrender the benefits that being ill or crippled affords. No illness, not even terminal cancer or AIDS, is totally devoid of benefits. Friends may be more considerate; one is the center of attention; get well cards and good wishes arrive; and any number of things accrue that do not ordinarily come to a healthy individual.

This explanation of cures does not detract from the wonder of the event. I don't mean to disparage anyone's religious faith, deny God's power, or diminish the mystical aura that surrounds these healing accomplishments. Every spring, when the crocuses and tulips come pushing up through the soil, I am awed. I understand about soil temperatures and the effect of lengthening hours of daylight, but this knowledge does not dampen the thrill of watching it all happen again.

CHAPTER ELEVEN

ON DOING NOTHING

MUCH OF THE PRESENT INSANITY that leads doctors to order unnecessary tests and to overtreat minor illnesses results from physicians, as a group, having little wisdom or judgment about *when to do nothing.* Presented with an ill patient, they direct their thoughts toward what to do, what tests to order, and what drugs to prescribe. Rarely does it occur to them that they may have already done too much, or that they should do nothing. Rarely will a physician tell a patient that he does not need medication because his problem will subside in a few days by itself. One of the hardest things for doctors to do is to wait, giving time for the medicines or the patient's natural recovery processes to work. And far too often, patients or their relatives demand immediate action. Few appreciate the wisdom of doing nothing. Perhaps television has taught us that all our problems can be solved in the forty or so minutes of drama we call a televised hour – and has affected our lives in other ways we have yet to consider. In any case, we generally expect immediate results.

When I first started practice, I contracted measles. I had assumed I'd had measles as a child, but there I was, with a fever of 104, covered with red spots. My three-year-old daughter walked into the bedroom, plopped a bouquet of dandelions on my chest, and said, "Here are some flowers, Daddy. Now get up!" In her three years of observation, she had noticed that receiving flowers appeared to be the key to immediate recovery.

The concept of doing nothing does not include abandoning the internal psychological work of talking to your bio-consciousness. This should be an ongoing conversation when you are ill, despite the medical treatment you may be receiving. The instructions to your autonomous reflex system must be clear and unequivocal, and it may even be a good idea to write them down and read them to yourself. Your efforts will augment the things your doctor does in your behalf.

Trained as we are to trust implicitly the decisions of our doctors, we rarely call a halt to treatment or forbid elaborate medical procedures to be performed. I recall a time in medical school when I attended a surgical conference. The chief resident presented an elderly man with a cancer of his ascending colon. The patient had already been placed on the surgical schedule for the next week. The man was slightly anemic but had no other problems referable to his tumor. Originally, he had come to the clinic in mild congestive heart failure secondary to arteriosclerosis and the anemia. A subsequent medical workup revealed the presence of the tumor.

The surgery department head, Dr. Warren H. Cole, asked the amphitheater full of students, residents, and professors what they felt should be done for the man. Everyone came up with a surgical plan of some sort. Then Dr. Cole asked for a show of hands of all the people who felt they should do nothing. Not a single hand went up. Finally, Dr. Cole raised his hand and said, "I do." Everyone in the amphitheater gasped. Dr. Cole stated that, with the tumor where it was, the man might live several more years with no treatment of any kind other than some iron tablets to treat his anemia. He pointed out that, because of his heart condition, the man was not a good surgical risk for an extensive operation. One of the professors of surgery said, "But the man has a cancer!" Dr. Cole responded by saying that his cancer would not kill him for many months and that he had no desire to kill the poor fellow on Thursday morning on the operating table with a knife, regardless of the good intent. Everyone got the point. The old man was discharged with some iron tablets for his anemia and given an outpatient appointment in three months. Dr. Cole was a great surgeon and a great teacher.

In general, doctors are not taught to make decisions in terms of limiting their efforts. On the contrary, once they establish that a problem exists and have defined its nature, they proceed to do "everything possible" to rectify the situation. In some instances, this is proper, but as in the case of the old man and the colon cancer, there are many times when this approach is most inappropriate. It is exactly these situations in which you, as a patient, must be ready to assert your own wishes, modifying the course of what is being proposed. If you really don't want "everything done," it is vital that your wishes be made known. A couple of generations ago, "doing everything" did not amount to much. Medical technology has changed that, and it is now possible to do things that were inconceivable then. *But just because we can do a thing is not reason alone to do it.* In fact, it is doubtful that a seriously ill patient could survive all the tests that could be run.

I recall a doctor in our clinic who admitted an elderly man to the hospital with his second massive stroke. The first had left him paralyzed on the left side but able to talk. He adjusted fairly well to his life in a nursing home, playing checkers and cards with the other residents. Then the fellow had a stroke on the other side, leaving him totally paralyzed, unable to speak or communicate. The man could swallow, but he refused to do so, for he wished to die rather than live in that condition. His doctor presented the case to our Monday morning conference, and stated that she intended to ask the surgeon to insert a stomach tube because the man refused to eat or drink. I voiced the opinion that she should leave the poor man alone. She responded, "What do you want me to do – play God? I can't leave him to die." I countered that playing God was exactly what she was attempting to do. I said, "God said, 'You had another stroke and it's time to die.' What you are saying is, 'No, God, You don't know what You're doing. I'm going to save this man.'" The doctor proceeded to have a stomach tube inserted, but, despite her extraordinary efforts, the fellow managed to die a couple of weeks later.

Just the other day, I was told of a recent case in a hospital in which an elderly man in his mid-eighties was admitted, dying of leukemia. His kidneys had failed, and he was in uremia. He also had several other things wrong with him, any one of which was imminently fatal. He had been under treatment for his leukemia for years, but at this point, he had too many problems to survive. With the help of his physician, he had weathered his illness for a long time, but now it was the moment to die. Finally, his heart stopped, putting a swift and painless end to many years of struggle with his leukemia.

Much to the dismay of the nursing staff, his doctor was determined to "save" him, and proceeded to do a full code on the poor man. This consisted of over an hour of external cardiac massage, numerous electroshocks to the heart, intubation, and a respirator, plus multiple injections of various heart drugs. The patient went ahead and died, but not before the doctor had run up several thousands of dollars in hospital charges, not to mention the fee for his services. It is in situations such as these that the relatives, or the patient if he or she is able, should *demand* that the doctor cease his efforts.

These are not isolated situations. All over the United States, as well as in other countries, dying people are being physically assaulted under the guise of attempting to resuscitate them or keep them alive a little longer. Often, dead bodies are subjected to resuscitative measures when they are brought to the emergency room, death having occurred at home or on the way to the hospital. The reason for this insanity is a misguided attempt to save lives. Another motive is the fear of a lawsuit if the hospital and doctor do not attempt to revive the person. In my opinion, one of the most insane activities we have promoted is teaching people to perform external cardiac massage.

One study documented the outcome of cardiac resuscitations on people over the age of seventy who were in the hospital at the time their hearts stopped. When patients' hearts stop while they are in the hospital, there is a better chance to resuscitate them than when the arrest occurs outside the hospital, since they receive attention more quickly. Well over seven hundred cases were included in the study. The patients received all the benefits of modern medicine. Every skill was directed toward getting their hearts beating again. Some of the patients were coded two and three times before finally managing to die. Out of those seven hundred plus individuals, nine people lived to go home after their cardiac arrest. Eight others survived but sustained irreversible brain damage and had to be placed in nursing homes. Statistically, the chance of any of those survivors living more than a year longer was nil. If we had a better understanding of life and death, we all would be in a better position to make judgments concerning resuscitation attempts.

Many doctors argue that to "save" nine people and have them return home was a victory and well worth the trouble and expense. Was it? Assume the average cost of doing a code, plus the doctor's fee, is around $3,000. Assuming only one code had been done on each patient, approximately $2,100,000 was spent in order for those nine people to live perhaps another year. That rounds out to over $230,000 for each person who made it home. To me, this is atrocious.

Try to respond to the following question without guilt or emotion coming into play, and imagine that it applies to you or a loved one: *Would there be a significant difference to you or your family if you died today or two weeks or two months from today?* I seriously doubt it. From a strictly economic point of view, we cannot afford to squander health care dollars so foolishly, spending millions on inappropriate procedures just to be able to say, "We did all we could." There is, after all, a limit to our resources. We must decide how we wish to spend them. I do not propose we cease treating elderly individuals. But I do think we need to evaluate each case and weigh the potential benefits of costly procedures that may have limited effects.

Do not misunderstand me here. There are times when the allopathic doctor will inform her patient she has nothing further to offer in the form of treatment that has any chance of curing the illness. Diseases such as terminal cancer, rheumatoid arthritis, multiple sclerosis, and others usually present this situation at some time in the course of the disease. Not being offered any alternative course of action, and trusting the wisdom of the doctor, it is then that patients sometimes ask for a medication that will put a final stop to the suffering. I do not believe that assisting in suicide is a proper role for the physician. We need to be very careful deciding that death is the only way out and that a patient needs to die right now. After all, when a person wishes to die, he or she can – and will. Keep in mind that plans arranged in Framework II are made for a reason and that protracted illnesses serve some valid purpose. So we need to be cautious about stepping in and radically altering the situation. In my opinion, administering an overdose of some chemical designed to end life is rarely an appropriate way out of the situation.

Of course, doctors should give dying patients enough medicine to keep them comfortable. I have seen instances in which doctors denied terminally ill patients who were in constant pain enough medicine to make them comfortable. The doctors justified this by saying they did not want the patient to become addicted to the pain medicine. I, too, have given patients with terminal cancer doses of narcotics adequate to relieve their pain, knowing that in a day or two they will develop the pneumonia that will end their life. A doctor is there, first, to help her patients recover more quickly if that is their goal, and then, to ease their pain and discomfort at the time of death.

Sometimes, help for the terminally ill is accomplished by simply letting the patient know that it is all right to die. The following true anecdote seems appropriate here. One of my friends confided that a relative was in the end stages of diabetes; she had lost one leg, her kidneys were failing, and she was in a coma following a heart attack. She had been in the hospital almost a month and was at a medical standstill. In spite of constant testing and continually changing medicines, nothing her doctor did seemed to make any difference. My friend went on to say that the family was exhausted, taking turns staying with her day and night. He said that her daughters talked to the woman, pleading constantly with her to wake up, to get well, and not to leave them.

I asked him how he got along with his relative. He replied that he had always liked her and they had gotten along quite well. I suggested that she might simply be waiting for permission to die. I proposed that he go into the room sometime when no one else was about and simply tell her it was all right to die and that she should not listen to her children; he should assure the woman that her daughters would adjust to her death and that everything would be fine. Later, my friend told me he had done just that. After he talked to her, he went to the cafeteria and had a cup of coffee. He returned thirty minutes later to find a nurse pulling the sheet over his relative's head.

This example of a death is not unique. If we only had a different and more realistic concept of what life and death mean, then situations such as these would be recognized almost daily. The death of my friend's relative was a beautiful event. Both of them knew her death was appropriate. My friend liked her and did not wish to see her suffer any longer. The fact that she died indicated that she was ready, it was time, and it was the thing to do. As it turned out, it seems that she was simply waiting to be told it was also all right.

One factor operating in this situation was that the doctor obviously did not know when to stop and let nature take its course. When I first began practice, I was taking care of an elderly lady who was in a nursing home. She was very senile and did not even recognize her son when he came to visit. In my zealousness to do everything, I had prescribed a number of fairly expensive medicines, totally convinced that she needed them all. Months dragged on, and her son, who was not wealthy, was feeling the financial pinch. He asked if there were not some medicines that could be discontinued. It had not occurred to me that she might not need them. Upon his suggestion, I went over the list in my mind and stopped them all save the digoxin for her heart. I informed the son that doing so might contribute to her dying. He assured me that he understood she was in a vegetative state and was essentially dead already. She lived another six months.

I recall a time in my training when we had a desperately ill woman on whom we had done a major surgical procedure. She was not responding as we hoped, and there was a frantic period in which we ordered many tests, changed medications, and obtained numerous X rays. It was about 1 A.M. when the attending surgeon suddenly said, "Let's stop. We have done enough. Now we need to give things time to work." The remainder of the night was most difficult for us. We sat and fidgeted, several in the team chain-smoked, we tried to make small talk, we drank coffee, and we paced the nurses' station. Finally, about 6 A.M., the patient began to show definite signs of improvement. Unfortunately, many physicians have not learned the discipline of doing nothing; they never cease ordering tests and changing medicines.

It is in exactly these situations when you, the patient or family member, empowered by your innate good sense, need to call a halt to the insanity. Relatively few situations are so dire that a few hours can't be spent in thoughtful consideration of the situation. After all, recovery from illness or injury ultimately lies in the patient's hands. The doctor should be considered as an adjunct to her patients' internal efforts to recover or remain in health. Once this principle is fully grasped, you may be less inclined to pressure your doctor to change medicines and order further tests.

CHAPTER TWELVE

A NEW PATH

I HAVE POINTED OUT that humankind is but a portion of a greater living entity we call the Universe. The Universe is intelligent consciousness and nothing more – as if that were not enough. In a very real way, the physical Universe is created by the manner in which we choose to observe it. And I've said that humans' range of perception is extremely narrow and limited, to the degree that we are incapable of appreciating the multidimensional nature of the Universe and of ourselves. In our incarnate state, we focus so intently upon those perceptions afforded us by our senses that we jump to the conclusion they are the only correct and valid views. We adhere to this position so firmly that, when presented with other ideas and solid evidence contrary to our beliefs, we reject them as impossible or, at best, unlikely.

Because of this intense focus of our egos, we have assumed a belief structure that views humanity as separate from the Universe. This outlook has led people who are coping with injury or disease to presume themselves the helpless victims of some terrible fate. All traditional medical approaches to treating illness are testimonies to that belicf. It must be said here that within these narrow, rigid constraints of belief, doctors have done marvelous things. I don't wish to diminish those accomplishments, but only to point out the futility of continuing along this path exclusively. At some point, unless there is a broadening of our concept of illness, medical progress will grind to a halt, for to deny the spiritual and multidimensional reality of humankind, as well as our own role in producing the very diseases from which we seek relief, is to court defeat in the long run.

What is the proper role of the physician? What should you expect, and what can you do to gain the most benefit should you become ill? In many ways, I have answered these questions throughout these pages. Each medical situation must, however, be assessed in light of its specific peculiarities. As has been shown, there is actually little need to eliminate many of the treatment modalities that are practiced today, but a different approach to their use must be taken and new priorities established. Certainly, you must come to realize, if you have not already, that there are many conditions allopathic doctors do not treat well or successfully. You must break the habit of turning automatically to traditional physicians for all the answers. Keep in mind a point that Dr. Andrew Weil makes in *Spontaneous Healing:* Allopathic doctors cannot cure cancer, degenerative diseases, or mental illness; they cannot effectively treat autoimmune diseases like multiple sclerosis, rheumatoid arthritis, and adult onset diabetes; they cannot properly manage psychosomatic diseases or treat viral infections. If you have one of these types of illness, you will probably be better off seeking help elsewhere.

The most significant medical advance of the next decade or so will be an opening of a new philosophy concerning the causes of disease and the most effective treatments. The new paradigm will dictate an altered approach to the timing and emphasis of the various methods and therapies to be applied. As a result, allopathy will no longer be thought of as the only respectable branch of medical care.

I had more than my share of trouble with the establishment over the forty-four years of my medical practice.

There were many things that I was not allowed to do because of the constraints placed upon me by my peers and the members of the clinic in which I practiced. But, within those boundaries, I was able to utilize many comprehensive approaches to my patients' illnesses. It was a difficult task politically, but, in the last years, I carried on a comprehensive, eclectic approach to my patients' illnesses in the midst of a group of conventional allopathic doctors. Some of my approach to diagnosis and my treatment modalities I kept secret. I frequently used hypnosis, performed a few chiropractic maneuvers, and applied kinesiology. I referred my patients to chiropractors, optometrists, and acupuncturists. I also consulted psychics from time to time for help in diagnoses. Patients with heart attacks were treated by the method outlined by Sodi-Pallares, using intravenous solutions of glucose, insulin, and potassium. With patients who cooperated, gave their support, and were unhelped by the standard approaches, *I obtained excellent results.*

What should you expect when you see a nontraditional doctor for the first time? Actually, the way he takes your medical history and does the physical examination should be similar to the way homeopaths are taught. The physician should converse with you in order to discover your beliefs, interests, goals, fears, habits, lifestyle, and the other psychosocial factors at work in your life. This process will lead to the questions of why you wished or allowed yourself to become ill, what the illness means to you, and what might be learned from it. If your doctor doesn't raise the issue, then ask the question of yourself. If he does not ask about your core beliefs regarding your health, pull up your old memories and start the discussion yourself. Ultimately, such information must come from your subconscious memories anyway. Then set about reinstructing yourself in healthier beliefs.

The person who develops a serious infection should be treated with the appropriate antibiotic. The individual with a peptic ulcer should be treated with the latest drugs. But, at the same time, the doctor should search out the underlying metaphysical cause of illness. For example, the newly discovered bacterium that is touted to be the cause of peptic ulcers is not *sufficient* cause for an ulcer to develop. People who do not have an ulcer often have the bacterium living in the lining of their intestinal tract. The bacterium can accomplish its work only with the cooperation of the individual who develops the ulcer. Or, more accurately, the patient who desires an ulcer seeks the active participation of the bacteria. These concepts need to be addressed in the process of health care. Every patient must comprehend his or her partnership in the formation of illness, and ultimately come to grips with the milieu of spiritual-physical interactions in which the illness was created.

Early in my practice, I had one family of patients whom I did not like. They were decent people, but they were dirty, unkempt, and troublesome, so I decided to treat them in such a way that they would not come back. The parents seemed to have little self-esteem and usually came to the office grimy and unwashed. I told the mother that her boys were dirty and that she ought to bathe them and clean them up. I lectured the parents about the way to raise a family. I was truly surprised when, instead of leaving, they began to change. They came to the office bathed and in clean clothes, and I sensed that they were developing some self-respect. They brought the kids in cleanly dressed and well scrubbed behind their ears. Over the years, they addressed everything that I had criticized about them. Time passed, and the children grew up, married, and raised kids of their own. The mother would bring pictures of them to show me. They had all turned out to be handsome, clean-cut young men with pretty, neatly dressed wives and good-looking children.

When I announced I was leaving the community, they came to my office crying and telling me how much I had meant to them and their family. They hugged me and thanked me for the concern I had shown throughout the years I had been their doctor. I found myself crying as well, for I had grown truly fond of them. Together we had worked out our differences and frustrations and had grown to love and respect one another. These good, honest, hardworking people taught me a lesson in human interaction. After that I drew closer to all of my patients and, as a result, learned to treat them more effectively.

Members of clinics, partnerships, or group practices not organized in such a way that patients can return to the same doctor visit after visit are deluding themselves if they believe that any doctor on staff is practicing preventive medicine or doing anything other than single-visit crisis intervention. Unless there is follow-up by the same doctor visit after visit, anything else is nigh to impossible. It is for these reasons that to obtain the best medical service, you should seek out the care of one doctor with whom you feel comfortable and with whom you are able to converse freely. *Don't choose hospital emergency rooms as a source for your primary care.*

If you are ill, no matter how seriously, and even if your doctor is not eclectic in his or her thinking, there is much you can do on your own. Work from the premise that you agreed to or sought the illness at some level. Does death appear attractive to you? If not death, what lesson are you attempting to teach yourself through the illness or injury? The lesson need not be great and profound. Remember, at times, a minor illness is used by the cellular consciousness as a means of sharpening its defenses. By simply going through the exercise of a psychological diagnosis, you can gain many insights about your disease and your well-being.

If you and your doctor are brave enough to implement the concepts described in this book, then there will be more to diagnosis and treatment than running tests and writing a few prescriptions. A bond of personal interaction will be established between you and your physician.

If your illness is heart disease, keep in mind that the doctor will not "save" you if at some deep spiritual level you intend to die. You must understand that, regardless of statistics, your survival is under your personal control; it will not be totally the result of the streptokinase, balloon angioplasty, or coronary bypass surgery. These treatments can, at times, be very helpful adjuncts to your recovery. They may well shorten your recovery time. But none of them is the final answer. Your eventual recovery is in your hands. You should take heed of the excellent results obtained by treating heart attacks by medical means, but to heal yourself, you need to go deeper.

When treatment of any disease is begun, it should include the *possibility* of employing all the standard treatments today along with other modalities. In the meantime, you should begin to instruct yourself in the mental attitude that will help in your recovery. Even if your doctor is not open to comprehensive beliefs, nothing prevents you from assuming these attitudes yourself. The two approaches are in no way contradictory. Indeed, they are complementary. You need to take an active role in the entire process, and the more involved you become, the better.

Even if you are merely susceptible to colds, the concepts addressed here will be helpful. There is no need to consult a doctor for an office call or a prescription. Your pharmacist can sell you some medicine that will be as effective as any the doctor can order and will save you the expense of an office visit. Meanwhile, you should spend some time trying to determine why you allowed yourself to be ill. What might you gain from being ill? What were you taught about the onset of colds by your parents?

Sit yourself down and begin thinking about all the colds you had when you were very young and what you were told about them. As you attempt to bring back these early memories, you will find that one memory leads to another, and your skill will improve with practice. Give yourself time to perfect your memory skills. It often takes a lot of practice. If you are unsuccessful doing this on your own, you might wish to consult a psychologist or a psychic. One of these professionals might hypnotize you and do some early life recall, helping you to remember your first cold. You might recall your mother admonishing herself for not properly covering you at night or for letting a draft in when she was bathing you. Perhaps you recall her telling you that going without your hat and mittens would surely make you sick.

Once these recollections are brought to consciousness, you alone, or with the help of the hypnotist, can address the problem and begin reinstructing your autonomous, reflexive ego system. Tell your autonomous system that, no matter how well intentioned, your mother's warnings were inappropriate and inaccurate. You can also instruct your immune system not to allow colds any longer. It may be that no connection can be found between your frequent colds and incidents or beliefs assumed early in this life. Your treating professional may then, using hypnosis or with the help of a psychic, discover some connection with another life in which a conditioned reflex was established, causing colds to develop when a certain set of circumstances occurs.

A personal event was quite instructive to me concerning how an inclusive approach to medical care can often solve the problems of chronic pain and disability. Beginning in the fall of 1988, I sustained a number of minor injuries to my right wrist. These all involved hammering or pounding with my right hand. About the time my wrist was beginning to recover from one episode, I would reinjure it.

By the spring of 1994, my wrist was swollen to half again its normal size, the ring and little fingers were curled into the palm of my hand, I could not hold a pen or a fork, the pain was more or less constant, and I had developed a burning pain from my neck down to my hand. I ate with my left hand. I wore a wrist brace and gritted my teeth as I typed my books. I took ibuprofen and went to my chiropractor, but neither helped. My wrist became more swollen and painful by the day. The burning pain running from my neck down my arm also grew worse. Since it was inconceivable that such minor injuries could account for over five years of continuous misery, I found, with the help of my friends Greg Satre and Ralph Warner, that I had sustained wrist and neck injuries that had led my bio-consciousness to maintain my pain. I knew then that it was necessary to free my bio-consciousness from whatever erroneous directions it was receiving.

Armed with a new understanding of my personal issues, which I'd gained through readings Greg and Ralph had given me, I started talking to myself, saying that *we* did not need the pain. I said that *our* body was new and different, and that *our* body had long since recovered from the injuries of digging holes, hammering on plumbing, and pounding clay. The effect was dramatic! Within forty-eight hours the swelling was gone and my neck, wrist, and hand were pain free. My fingers worked and my hand and wrist functioned normally! This example demonstrates the clear linkage between the mind and the bio-consciousness. It also illustrates the power of the mind to create, or sustain, illnesses and injuries. All this I can testify to from personal experience.

Of course, not everyone with a sprained wrist needs the help of a psychic or a hypnotist. In most instances, some over-the-counter medicine from the drugstore will serve the purpose. Even in the healing of an illness or injury that has persisted because of a connection to another life, it is not essential to be hypnotized or to have a psychic reading. It is only necessary for you to acknowledge the *possibility* of another life connection and then to go about reinstructing your autonomous reflex system. If there is no actual relationship with a previous life, the reinstruction will work anyway. On a recent television program called "Healing and the Heart," doctors had the courage to speak openly about cases in which there was no scientific explanation for the excellent results that had been documented. All the patients presented had been cured by nontraditional means. One case study was highly instructive, demonstrating how illness can be sought and cured by psychic means alone. It involved a woman who appeared to be in her early fifties. Both she and her husband were psychologists. The woman developed a cancer of her lung and opted not to have surgery or regular therapy of any kind. She did some soul searching and admitted that she had had an unresolved childhood trauma that resulted in her feeling unlovable despite her having a loving husband and children. Some of the interpretation I am about to give is little more than speculation, but the information on the program seemed to point clearly in this direction.

The woman stated that her lack of self-esteem was the problem that had resulted in her cancer. Her disease was in every sense a gift – a wake-up call – and at the same time a potential way out. If she was not going to deal with her trauma and resolve it, then there was little reason to continue this life. She and her husband tackled her childhood trauma, and she resolved it in her spirit. As she developed a new footing, she came to accept that she was, after all, worthy of her own love and respect as well as that of her family. What is more, she made the decision to live rather than to die. As a result of this, her lung cancer simply disappeared. The program showed the chest X rays before and after. There is no doubt of the cure.

She had been well and cancer free for eight years at the time the program was filmed.

This is an example of inclusive medicine at its best, but in this incident the patient did not need outside help. Being a psychologist, she had the necessary skills to work out her own problem, with the help of her husband. Doctors see and hear of these cases from time to time, but, because the examples fall outside their rigid belief system, they are ignored. Rather than learning from these wonderful people and their dramatic, spontaneous cures, too many doctors shake their heads in confusion, turn their backs, shut off their minds, and reject the whole experience, denying the validity of the case and even their own observations.

If the woman with the lung cancer had developed pneumonia that was threatening to kill her, a visit to the doctor for some antibiotics would have been appropriate. The doctor could use his knowledge concerning bacteriology and pharmacology to prescribe the right medicine and buy her some time. If her nutrition had been poor, a nutritionist could have prescribed vitamins and a better diet. On the other hand, for a doctor to have taken the woman into the hospital, surrounded her with associates and nurses programmed to believe that nearly all lung cancer patients die within a year, operated on her, and concluded he had done something wonderful would have been foolish and naive.

When I practiced medicine in Champaign, I had a fair number of Christian Scientists as patients. I had no trouble convincing them to take the medicine I prescribed. I explained that the medicine would not make them well, nor would it detract from their relationship with God. The medicine was no more than an adjunct to what they were already doing. The antibiotic might kill the bacteria that were causing the infection, but their bodies still had to get well. It is the same with surgery and drugs for any disease. There are occasions when doctors can buy patients time while the *real* healing process is taking place. If a person has a bowel obstruction caused by cancer of the colon, he will die within a week or so, without having an opportunity to reinstruct his bio-consciousness to eliminate the tumor. Surgery can relieve the obstruction and give him time to discover what is blocking his opportunity to fulfill his greatest constructive potential. If you develop appendicitis, without surgery the appendix will likely rupture and you will develop peritonitis. Even when treated with antibiotics, peritonitis has a considerable mortality rate. If you have appendicitis, you *need* an appendectomy. While you are under the anesthetic, the doctor can give you a number of suggestions that will hasten your recovery and make you more comfortable. But you should examine the underlying metaphysical reasons for the illness and what the event may have taught you.

It is well established that, except for common skin cancers and carcinoma in situ of the cervix, malignancy involving internal organs or the breast may never be a localized disease, and no amount of extensive surgery will "get it all." Many years ago, at the University of Illinois, Dr. Stewart Roberts did an experiment in which he drew blood from the arms of women with breast cancers while someone else examined the breasts that had the tumors. In every instance, Dr. Roberts demonstrated that the examination caused a shower of malignant cells to be released into the bloodstream. Obviously, then, survival from cancer does not depend upon surgery or drugs, but upon the patient's ability to defend against the malignant cells. We must come to grips with the fact that ultimate survival still depends upon the patient's controlling her cancer herself. Eclectic medicine and its various branches are simply geared toward augmenting the efforts of the body.

It has been known for years that bone fractures heal much more quickly if patients visualize their recovery while meditating. The doctor should tell each person to visualize his bone healing rapidly and then leave it up to the individual to create his own fantasy. A patient might visualize little elves laying down slabs of calcium like tiny bricks to span the fracture or picture the bone cells marching across the fracture site with buckets of calcium to fill the gap, making strong bridges of new bone.

The same technique is helpful in healing illnesses. Once an offending food is identified and eliminated, the person with multiple sclerosis can facilitate her recovery, perhaps by visualizing hundreds of repairmen wrapping new insulation around her nerve fibers. If you have an infection, you can imagine Pac-man® characters gobbling up the dead tissue and germs. It is of no importance how you choose to visualize the healing process. Such childlike, unscientific imagery does work, and it works by focusing the intent of the mind and imparting a clear message to the cells.

The individual who resents his injury or illness and spends much of his time glaring at his cast or his bottles of medicine, convinced that, with his bad luck, the fracture will not heal or he will remain sick, is very likely to take a long time in recovery. If you think these thoughts when you are ill or injured, you actually instruct your bio-consciousness to ignore its prime directive to mend the injury or cure the illness. We understand that our bodies are in a constant state of rebuilding. We must come to know, just as certainly, that we influence the healing of our diseases, wounds, broken bones, burns, and the like at all times.

About a year ago, Greg told me that he had tripped in his kitchen. In an attempt to catch himself, he put out his arm and accidentally thrust his hand into a large pan full of boiling hot grease. Immediately, he talked to his hand. He told his skin cells that they did not have to be burned, that they had too much work to do to be inconvenienced by burns and blisters.

212

He literally refused for his hand to be burned and so instructed his cells, telling them that they were all in good condition, telling them not to die, swell, or become inflamed. Within a second or two, the pain completely vanished and the skin appeared to be perfectly normal. The next day, his hand showed no sign of having been burned. Only one spot, near the back of his wrist, was red and had a small blister. He said that was the one place he had neglected to focus his attention as he mentally swept over his hand, giving his skin cells their instructions.

Since that conversation, I have been practicing the same thing. I do all the cooking in our home, and small burns are not uncommon. I told myself that if Greg could prevent being burned, I could do it too. It has been several months since I have allowed myself to be actually burned. I immediately talk to the area, telling it that it is all right, that there is no need to be burned. The pain promptly goes away and no sign of a burn develops. The last time this happened, a large amount of hot bacon grease had splashed on the back of my hand. I grabbed my hand, looked intently at it, and, without thinking, said, "You're all right." And it was. Then I realized that the grease had not even felt hot. As you see, these healing concepts are not just things I have read or heard about. On the contrary, they are events I have experienced myself and know to be true. The healing power of the psyche is available to everyone. You can experience it as well, if you set your mind to it.

It seems patently clear, at least to me, that everyone would benefit by entertaining the concepts in this book concerning the causes of illness and how to cure it. You are not a victim, but a willing participant and, more often than not, the author of your illnesses. I'm fully aware that I have repeated this statement many times, but it is such a critical element in the new paradigm for illness and recovery that it must be stressed at every opportunity.

Absolutely nobody is a victim of anything – not illness, not death, not the so-called misfortunes of life. Each of us is the creator of our physical and emotional environment and our total well-being. Consciously or unconsciously, we choose our participation in life at every stage and in every circumstance. And we have the power to shape those circumstances if only we will take it up.

If you had never heard of a common cold and knew nothing about the illness, you might well die of it – if you believed that you would. Every symptom would be frightening. You might imagine suffocating to death when your nose became clogged. As a matter of fact, this is a time of panic for an infant with her first cold. Upon finding it impossible to breathe freely through her nose, a baby often becomes frightened until she realizes that it is possible to breathe through her mouth. With no understanding of the nature of the disease, a person might not instruct his immune system to counter the effects of a cold virus. Fear and expectations of death might be thought of as directions to his bio-consciousness not to defend itself against the virus. Yes, it is possible that you could die from a head cold.

The same thing happens when an individual is diagnosed with cancer, AIDS, or any other fatal or serious disease. In the metaphor of this culture, a diagnosis of cancer or AIDS is synonymous with death. Aware that the medical profession does not have a real cure, and taking cues from individuals he has known with these diseases and from his doctor, the patient may program himself to die. As I have said, about the only instances in which doctors can cure cancer are *very* early stages of cervical cancer and basal cell carcinomas of the skin. There still is no effective treatment for AIDS.

Some modern drugs do kill cancer cells, and if an individual wishes to live, they can help her achieve that goal. But if she wishes to die, no therapy will be successful. If she seeks death and her means to accomplish this are thwarted by the cancer drugs, surgery, and radiation, she can always die of some side effect of the medicine or in another creative way. In any case, the person with a cancer has probably never been told that her body defends itself from a malignancy in much the same way it defends against infections. It likely never occurs to her that she can reverse the cancerous condition herself. She looks for help from without, seeking a better surgeon, a newer drug, a fancier hospital, a different piece of diagnostic equipment. Neither she nor her doctor thinks of her being an active participant in developing the disease or in the healing process. If she joins a cancer support group, more than likely she will be surrounded by well-meaning people who concentrate on coping with the disease and their inevitable death rather than on learning how to live and not die.

Doctors are vaguely aware of a thing called the will to live, but they don't truly comprehend how it works. By recognizing this phenomenon, they do give some credence to the ideas I have introduced. To my knowledge, no one has actually studied the will to live other than to describe the general personality type of people who seem to possess it. Every doctor who has been in practice for any period of time has seen at least one patient who refused to die of his illness in spite of the doctor's own learned predictions. Delighted that the patient has recovered, few doctors give it a second thought. But if they began to reason through these incidents, they would be faced with the same metaphysical questions considered here.

Throughout this book, I have introduced some concepts that many of you may consider radical or even unbelievable. I have said that matter is alive and has the ability to communicate, remember, think, and create. I have said that your cells have their own consciousness separate from your mind, with the desire to seek value fulfillment in their lives that takes the form of joyful cooperation with the vaster consciousness that is you. I have indicated that you plan your life, create your own body, and orchestrate your health or infirmities in a network of spiritual reality that represents the real Universe. I have said that you have total control over your recovery from the injuries and diseases you attract to your temporal existence. All of these statements are part of a way of perceiving life and the Universe different from the one to which we have previously committed ourselves. But their variance from the "normal" view of things does not make them less valid.

I wrote of taking you through the window of paradox from the room of conventional thought into the garden for a vaster perception of reality. As we walked through this philosophical garden, chapter by chapter, these truths were phrased in a straightforward manner with sentences that did not equivocate. This was done purposely for if any of this is to "work", the thoughts must not waver. The cellular consciousness picks up on the hesitation and implied doubt and fails to respond to what it considers to be an intellectual exercise of sorts, a rambling of the mind.

I have made many references to multiple incarnations and the fact that memories from other lives can bleed through into your subconscious thoughts and affect your recovery from some present illness or injury. I know from personal experience, in addition to observations when working with numerous patients, that this is true. However, if you are still uncertain of the truth of multiple incarnations, it will be helpful for you to assume a neutral stance on the teeter-totter of assumption and at least acknowledge the possibility that these concepts are true. My personal belief is that recovery from every injury or illness is effected by all life experiences, whether or not one believes that some of those experiences occurred in another existence. I have done everything short of promise you that a cure can be obtained through these unconventional concepts and understanding. And you *can* heal yourself. But there is a catch to it. To be successful, these concepts must become far more than an intellectual exercise with which to play the next time you sprain your ankle, burn your hand, or catch a cold. For any of this to be successful, you must believe it with all your might, right down to your toes. For it to work, there can be absolutely no doubts, however slight or insignificant you may believe them to be. This is why I have stressed the importance of having unequivocal focused intent. Half believing will not work. Trying it for fun will only be an exercise in futility, and you may conclude that I have, after all, written a book of nonsense or a fairy tale.

For you to be successful in your self-healing efforts, it is critical for you to know such healings are possible. Such an understanding requires that you *completely* restructure your belief system, casting out all previously held notions concerning the causes of illness. Throughout your life you have been told, in one way or another, that self-healing is not reasonable and that you must consult a doctor for all illnesses and injuries other than very minor ones. To counter this, it is usually necessary to say to yourself repeatedly that self-healing is a fact and that you can in reality, accomplish it. Again, do not equivocate when giving yourself – your autonomous reflex system – the new instructions. Your bio-consciousness takes instructions and thoughts literally, so word your statements clearly and decisively. It may be helpful for you to write out your affirmations – your instructions to your autonomous reflex system – and read them each time. Doing so will ensure that the wording is forceful and unequivocal and that you leave nothing out.

If, after this warning, you are intent upon developing your own abilities in some of these areas, it is important not to "try." Trying is not doing. Even the word "try" has the hidden implication of failure. Consider the difference between trying

217

to raise your arm and raising it. Approach your healing with confidence and total belief in the concepts, knowing that you can accomplish what others do.

Should you be involved in a treatment program for cancer, you are already deeply imbedded in the allopathic approach to treatment. Since you have, no doubt, bought into that approach, it is unlikely that the concepts introduced here will be of more than passing interest. If, however, you are interested in augmenting the effect of the drugs and radiation, here is some practical information you must consider. Most anticancer drugs are very toxic. Each one is capable of killing every cell in your body, cancerous or not. The theory is to kill the cancer cells while not quite killing you. As a result, your cells are so poisoned by the medicines that they may not be in any condition to heal themselves while you are under therapy. For this reason, all your intent, no matter how focused and pure it may be, may not do much good. Wait until the doctor has taken you off the medicine or you are between courses. Then, the principles given here may be successful. Linus Pauling, for example, has indicated that massive doses of vitamin C to treat cancer are more effective if the patient has not received chemotherapy. You will recall that Greg Satre and the psychologist with the lung cancer opted not to have any form of conventional therapy. Except for the cancer growing within them, their bodies were healthy and capable of responding to their mental commands.

If you are ill and seem to be getting well from the treatment you are receiving from your doctor, ***do not stop your treatment***. You believed it would help or you would not have gone to the physician in the first place. Remember, all treatments are effective if the patient believes they are. If it is your subconscious intention to get well, you will, and nothing will alter that.

I hope that the concepts in this book will be applied by those who are not ill and wish to remain healthy. They should also prove vital to individuals with chronic pain and nonfatal illnesses. Even if you have a deadly condition, no harm will come by adopting these ideas as your belief system, and you may be gratified at the results. When you truly understand the tenets of this book and adopt them with conviction, your life will become all the proof you need.

Author's Page

O.T. Bonnett is a retired physician, a published author, and a sculptor. He was born in 1925 in Salina, Kansas and grew up in Kansas, Wyoming and Illinois. He graduated from University of Illinois College of Medicine in 1948. After his internship and two years of general surgery residency, he was activated into the Navy during the Korean war, serving for two years. The first eighteen months he was attached to the Second Marine Division at Camp LeJeune, North Carolina, and the last six months he was in charge of a thirty bed surgical ward at the U.S. Naval hospital there.

Following military service, he entered general practice in Champaign-Urbana, Illinois. He practiced eighteen years as a solo practitioner, delivering babies, performing major surgery, and all the things associated with being a general practitioner. In the fall of 1970, he joined The Bellaire Medical Group, an HMO based in the coal fields of West Virginia and Ohio where he served as Chief of the Department of Adult Medicine. In 1987 he left active practice and assumed a position as Medical Director of Miners Colfax Hospital in Raton, New Mexico. He retired after five years and began writing books.

In the fall of 1987 while exhibiting his sculpture at an art show in Denver, he met Greg Satre who had a pottery booth next to him. He says their meeting was one of the most significant events of his life, ranking with his birth, graduating from medical school, and meeting his spirit guide, Pan.

Throughout his entire life, he has been interested in philosophy and metaphysics. As a boy, he read Emerson and Lao Tse. Many metaphysical principles were incorporated into his practice. Some fifty years ago, through the use of hypnosis, he learned that we all experience multiple incarnations. This knowledge, coupled with metaphysical principles, was helpful in the recovery of many patient's illnesses and injuries.

Dr. Bonnett published two scientific articles: Effects of Positive Suggestion on Surgical Patients and The Treatment and Prevention of Acute Dysionic Myocardial Necrosis. In addition, he is the author of three published books: *Reincarnation: The View from Eternity, What I Learned After*

Medical School (formerly titled Confessions of a Healer) and *Why Healing Happens.*

The first forty-five years of his life, he was deeply involved with the Presbyterian church. He attended Sunday school and church regularly and was an elder for many years. Various experiences led him to adopt a different stance in life.

He and his wife, Hazel, live in Raton, New Mexico with their two cats, Barney and Zoro. Their home is as ancient 125 year old dwelling which they remodeled and redecorated, doing much of the work themselves. He enjoys the solitude and the wide expanse of the eastern slope of the Rocky Mountains where bear and deer are frequent visitors to his yard, not to mention the many species of birds that come to his feeders.

O.T. Bonnett
PO Box 1272
Raton, NM 87740
(505) 445-2847
BONNETT12345@MSN.COM

Other Books Published by Ozark Mountain Publishing, Inc.

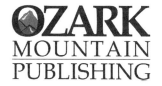

Notes